Table of Contents

Table of Contents	1
Questions	3
MACE	3
Answers	52

About Dynamic Path

Dynamic Path has a simple mission statement: To help you pass your test and get ahead by providing high-quality study questions. Whether you're preparing for a real estate agent licensure or an AP exam, we want to help you succeed.

We believe in our content, and we offer 50 free practice questions for each of our exams on our site. You can take a sample test or study session with us online, and get the results emailed to you.

All exam modules are written and edited by experts in their field, and each practice question is accompanied by a detailed explanation.

There are several ways to learn with Dynamic Path. You can browse exams and learn on the site or through our mobile apps, available for iOS, Mac, Android, Kindle, and Windows.

Dynamic Path is a product of Upward Mobility, a 100% woman- and minority-owned company (SOWMBA-certified) based in Boston, MA. It was formed to create free and low-cost high-quality education and test preparation material that is witty, engaging, and adds value to the learning process. You can learn more about our social mission and values here, or read a message from one of our co-founders here. You can also learn more about our staff here.

If you have any questions, suggestions, or technical problems, feel free to email us at support@dynamicpath.com.

Happy studying!

Questions

MACE

1. **For which of the following life-threatening adverse effects is it MOST important to ensure that you have obtained informed consent? The patient has been prescribed lovastatin (Mevacor/Altocor).**

    A. Asthenia
    B. Pruritis
    C. Rhabdomyolysis
    D. Lupus-like syndrome

2. **A 72 year old woman has been prescribed Boniva. What is the best way for this prescription to be taken?**

    A. Right before bedtime.
    B. With minimum water and in the evening at least two hours after a meal
    C. Anytime during the day with no food requirements
    D. In the morning at least 30 minutes before any meal and with a full glass of water.

3. **A patient arrives and asks you about his Depacon prescription. Which of the following is important to determine and why?**

    A. Whether the patient takes Clonazepam and has a history of absence seizure, because these may increase with Depacon.
    B. Whether the patient drinks alcohol, because alcohol increases the CNS depressive effect blood concentration of valproate.
    C. Both A and B are correct.
    D. Neither A nor B are correct.

4. **Which of the following is the correct epinephrine dosage with an infusion rate of 30 mL/hr and an epinephrine concentration of 1 mg in 250 mL of a solution of 5% dextrose in water?**

    A. 2 mcg/min
    B. 4 mcg/min
    C. 10 mcg/min
    D. 135 mcg/min

5. **Which of the following drugs is a beta-adrenergic blocker?**

    A. Busiperone
    B. Budenoside
    C. Bisoprolol
    D. Phenoxybenzamine

6. **Which of the following is the correct nitroglycerin dosage with an infusion rate of 9 mL/hr and a nitroglycerine concentration of 50 mg in 250 mL of a solution of 5% dextrose in water (D$_5$W)?**

    A. 30 mcg/min
    B. 60 mcg/min
    C. 25 mcg/min
    D. 100 mcg/min

7. **Which of the following creams reduces contraceptive effectiveness?**

    A. Clindamycin
    B. Vagifem
    C. Miconazole
    D. Metronidazole

8. **Which of the following should be used on a short-term basis due to the risk of physical and psychological dependence?**

    A. Sustiva
    B. Edrophonium
    C. Ambien
    D. None of the above; these are all very safe medications.

9. **Your patient has a prescription for Glucophage/metformin (850 mg three times a day (TID)). His doctor added Glyburide to increase glycemic control. What is the maximum dose of metformin in combination with another hypoglycemic?**

    A. 1000 mg TID
    B. 2000 mg every day
    C. Nothing; they cannot be combined.
    D. Whatever dose is needed to reduce blood sugar to below 126 mg/dL.

10. **Which of the following vitamins is water-soluble?**

    A. Vitamin E
    B. Vitamin D
    C. Vitamin K
    D. Vitamin B_{12}

11. **For which of the following pediatric conditions has the FDA (Food and Drug Administration) approved the use of decongestants?**

    A. Allergic rhinitis and the common cold, for children over the age of 2.
    B. Sinusitis and allergic rhinitis, for children over the age of 5.
    C. Sinusitis, rhinitis and the common cold, for children over the age of 12.
    D. Sinusitis for any child.

12. **A patient on phenelzine (Nardil; 15 mg tablets) asks you if there is any food he should avoid. You can tell him:**

    A. There is no problem; you can eat anything you want.
    B. You should stay away from peanut butter.
    C. You should stay away from high fat foods because it decreases absorption of the drug.
    D. Any foods with tyramine should be avoided.

13. **A patient is diagnosed with iron-deficiency anemia and is give iron supplements. They ask if they should take it with food. Your response is:**
    A. Iron is best absorbed when taken with milk.
    B. Iron should be taken with food to increase absorption and minimize gastric upset.
    C. Iron is best taken with water only and at least one hour before eating.
    D. None of the above is correct.

14. **Which are the most serious adverse effects associated with Lithium?**
    A. Hepatitis
    B. Stevens-Johnson Syndrome
    C. Sinus node dysfunction
    D. None of the above

15. **Which of the following drugs would be likely to be used in an elderly patient with hypertension? The patient doesn't remember the name of the pill, and only remembers that it is a pretty little pink, oval pill, and she is certain it is not one of those "water pills." Which of the following is most likely her medication?**
    A. 0.5 mg alprazolam/Xanax
    B. 80 mg/12.5 mg Diovan HCT
    C. 500 mg Amoxil
    D. 200 mg Augmentin

16. **Which of the following vitamins are excreted in the urine?**
    A. Vitamin A
    B. Vitamin B_2
    C. Vitamin E
    D. Vitamin D

17. **A patient of yours is on tegaserod. Which of the following co-morbidities would indicate a need for caution?**
    A. Alzheimer's Disease
    B. Gallstone
    C. Concurrent viral infections
    D. Pre-existing cataracts

18. **A patient comes to you in her 3rd trimester and says that she forgot to tell you about one of her medications; it is trandolapril. She is now concerned about the safety of her unborn child. What can you tell her?**
    A. If the doctor prescribed it, it is safe.
    B. Trandolapril is contraindicated during pregnancy. We will find a substitute for you while you are pregnant.
    C. There is no contraindication to taking Trandolapril while pregnant.
    D. Trandolapril is contraindicated for women who are breastfeeding, but not for women who are pregnant.

19. **Which of the following is a combination of amlodipine and benzepril?**

    A. Premphase
    B. Vusion
    C. Truvada
    D. Lotrel

20. **Which of the following has a "black box warning" associated with it?**

I. Parenteral tobramycin
II. Gadolimium-based contrast agents
III. Topical tacrolimus
IV. Salmeterol

    A. I and II only
    B. II and III only
    C. All have black box warnings associated with them
    D. None of the listed agents have black box warnings associated with them.

21. **A clinic specializing in congestive heart failure has asked you to monitor outcomes on a number of elderly patients. They use both nesiritide and tezosentin and would like your input on these drugs. You can tell them:**

    A. Tezosentin is an endothelin-receptor dual agonist but has been shown to be ineffective in improving dyspnea or reducing the risk of cardiovascular events.
    B. Nesiritide is a recombinant human B-type natriuretic peptide and should not be used in patients with low cardiac filling pressures.
    C. Both A and B are correct.
    D. A is correct, but B is incorrect. The filling pressure may safely be less than 90mm Hg as long as the patient is continuously monitored.

22. **A patient has a prescription for lansoprazole. What is the likely diagnosis?**

I. GERD
II. Duodenal ulcer
III. Crohn's disease
IV. UC

    A. I and III are likely diagnoses
    B. I and II are likely diagnoses
    C. III and IV are likely diagnoses
    D. Lansoprazole is not used in any of these conditions.

23. **A patient is taking Nimotop (nimodopine) 60 mg PO q 4hrs. Nimotop is available as a 30 mg capsule. The label reads: Take two capsules 2 times a day with meals. What is the error on the label?**
    A. The capsules should be taken every 4 hours.
    B. The capsule should never be taken by mouth.
    C. The capsules should not be taken except 1 hour before meals or 2 hours after meals
    D. None of the above

24. **As a medication assistant, you are given an order that reads: Hydromorphone, 80 mg, PO q 4hrs. What is wrong with this order?**
    A. It represents an overdose.
    B. It is correct as written for severe pain.
    C. Hydromorphone is only given by injection.
    D. Hydromorphone is only given as a rectal suppository.

25. **You are asked to monitor a multiple myeloma patient on IV melphalan. Which of the following lab parameters need to be determined to appropriately monitor the patient?**
    A. Serum glucose levels.
    B. Creatinine clearance.
    C. Serum potassium levels
    D. Platelet counts

26. **Which of the following warnings are appropriate for tetracycline?**
I. Do not take antacid with tetracycline
II. Do not take with milk to avoid stomach upset.
III. Avoid sunlight.
IV. If prolonged therapy is anticipated, regular blood testing will be required.
    A. I and II only
    B. II and III only
    C. III only
    D. All are true.

27. **A patient is taking 40 mg PO of simvastatin with her evening meal. She comes to you to ask about what she read on the Internet about adverse effects, saying that for the last 2-3 weeks, her legs felt like they were cramping. Which of the following tests would you recommend?**
    A. Liver function tests
    B. A CBC (complete blood count) and a full Comp Metabolic (chemistries) test
    C. Total simvastatin urine concentrations
    D. Creatine phosphokinase (CPK), the MM isoenzyme.

28. **Of the following terms is another term for Vitamin K?**

I. **Mephyton**
II. **Phytonadione**
III. **Pyridoxine**

    A. I only
    B. I and II only
    C. All three are terms for Vitamin K.
    D. None of the three listed are terms for Vitamin K.

29. **A patient using minocycline approaches you asking what possible side effects there might be. What could you tell him?**

I. **Hemolytic anemia**
II. **Pericarditis**
III. **Dental problems**

    A. I only
    B. II only
    C. II and III only.
    D. All are possible side effects.

30. **Which of the following medications would be appropriate to treat a *Candida* infection in a child of 12 years?**

    A. Tobramycin
    B. Fluconozole
    C. Ampicillin
    D. Clindamycin

31. **What is the most common and most serious adverse effect of sulindac (Clinoril)?**

I. **GI bleeding**
II. **Hyperkalemia**
III. **Hyponatremia**

    A. I only
    B. II and III only
    C. I and II only
    D. III only

32. **Which of the following would be best considered for the treatment of acute migraines?**

    A. Loxapine
    B. Etanercept
    C. Sumatriptan
    D. Eptifibatide

33. **For which of the following conditions would QVAR be indicated?**

I. COPD
II. Community acquired pneumonia
III. Asthma

    A. I only
    B. II only
    C. III only
    D. I and II only

34. **A patient is on simvastatin. What is the biochemical pathway that is inhibited by this drug?**

    A. The pentose phosphate pathway
    B. The mevalonate pathway
    C. The eiconosoid pathway
    D. The electron transport chain

35. **Saquinavir is used to treat _____ and is contraindicated with/in _____.**

    A. Infection with Gram (+) bacteria, blood dyscrasias
    B. Mycoplasma, immunosuppresion
    C. Advanced HIV infections, concurrent use of anti-arrhythmics
    D. Viral URIs, emphasema

36. **Eletriptan (Relpax) is used to treat _____, and it is contraindicated with/in _____. Its major adverse reaction is _____.**

    A. Gout, blood dyscrasias, arrhythmias
    B. Rheumatoid arthritis, osteoporosis, spontaneous fractures.
    C. Diabetes, hypoglycemia, respiratory arrest
    D. Migraine (with or without aura), uncontrolled hypertension, ischemia

37. **Which of the following statements is false concerning Phase I, II or III clinical trials?**

    A. A phase I trial is often quite large (N>500) and seeks to determine the safe dose range for a new drug.
    B. A phase II trial is often larger than a phase I trial and seeks to determine if a new drug is effective enough to test in a phase III trial and to delineate adverse effects.
    C. A Phase III trial compares a new treatment with an established treatment and is usually much larger than either a phase I or a phase II trial.
    D. All three of the statements are correct.

38. **A patient is prescribed Roferon-A. Of the following, what is the most likely diagnosis?**

    A. A MRSA infection
    B. Multiple sclerosis
    C. Chronic hepatitis C
    D. Infertility.

39. **Of the following medications, which is NOT used to treat Hashimoto's Thyroiditis?**

    A. Levothyroxing
    B. Propylthiouracil
    C. Cytomel
    D. Thyrolar

40. **Of the following organisms, which would be susceptible to azithromycin?**

    I. Chlamydia pneumoniae
    II. Staphyloccoccus pneumoniae
    III. Mycoplasma hominis

    A. I and II only
    B. I, II and III
    C. I and III only
    D. I only

41. **A patient that is newly diagnosed with multiple sclerosis (MS) is concerned about the interferon-beta injections she was told to give herself. What would you want to make her aware about concerning adverse reactions?**

    I. The most common adverse reactions involve the injection site and include pain, redness and soreness.
    II. Keep the syringe in the refrigerator, rotate the areas where you inject and use NSAIDS for any flu-like symptoms.
    III. The most serious adverse reactions concern suicidal ideation, cardiac arrhythmias, blood abnormalities and intestinal obstruction.

    A. Both I and II are correct
    B. Both II and III are correct
    C. Only I and III are correct
    D. All are correct

42. **Which of the following is the brand name for rifabutin?**

    A. Sandimmune
    B. Neoral
    C. Mycobutin
    D. Gengraf

43. **Which of the following disorders is a contraindication for the use of sulindac?**

    A. Asthma
    B. A history of breast cancer
    C. Cardiac arrhythmias
    D. G6PD (Glucose-6-Phosphate Dehydrogenase) deficiency

44. **Concerning ulcerative colitis (UC) and Crohn's disease (CD), which of the following statements is TRUE?**

I. Ulcerative colitis (UC) is a risk factor for colon cancer.
II. Crohn's disease (CD) can appear anywhere from the mouth to the rectum.
III. UC has a continuous pattern of GI inflammation.
IV. CD has a segmented pattern of GI inflammation.

    A. I and II only
    B. II and IV only
    C. III and IV only
    D. All are true

45. **Which of the following statements accurately reflects the difference between accuracy and precision in measurements?**

I. Precision is a measure of how close an experimental value is to the dependent variable.
II. Accuracy is a measure of how close an experimental value is to the expected value.
III. Precision is a measure of how close a series of experimental values are to each other.
IV. Accuracy is a measure of how close an experimental value is to the independent variable.

    A. I and II are true.
    B. II and III are true.
    C. I and IV are true.
    D. II and III are true.

46. **A patient has a Glucose-6-Phosphate Dehydrogenase (G6PD) deficiency. Of the following drugs, which should be avoided in this patient?**

    A. Macrolides
    B. Omeprazole
    C. Vitamin B_{12}
    D. Quinolones

47. **Which of the following is a common anti-emetic used as an adjunct in chemotherapy AND is a 5HT3 receptor antagonist?**

    A. Aprepitant
    B. Ondansetron
    C. Metoclopramide
    D. All of the above.

48. **Which of the following is TRUE of HIPAA (Health Insurance Portability and Accountability Act)?**

I. One purpose was to improve the Medicare and Medicaid programs
II. It is enforced by the Office of Civil Rights
III. HIPAA regulations apply to electronic healthcare transactions
IV. HIPAA addresses privacy issues as one of its primary goals.

    A. Only answer IV is true
    B. Only answers II and IV are true
    C. Only answers I, II and IV are true
    D. All the answers are true

49. **Which of the following can induce a photoreaction in a sensitive individual?**

I. Chlorthiazide
II. Oxaprozin
III. Tretinoin
IV. Hydroxyurea

    A. I and II only
    B. I and IV only
    C. I, II and III only
    D. III only

50. **Rivastigmine is a(n) _____ used to treat _____ and rarely has the adverse effect of inducing _____.**

    A. ACE inhibitor, hypotension, tachycardia
    B. Voltage-gated Na^+ channel blocker, hypertension, aplastic anemia
    C. Cholinesterase inhibitor, Alzheimer's disease, anxiety and tremor
    D. Serotonin antagonist, post-operative nausea and vomiting, hyperemesis

51. **Ribavarin is a _____ used to treat _____ that rarely has the adverse effect of inducing _____.**

    A. Serotonin antagonist, nausea and vomiting, paralysis
    B. Voltage-gated Na^+ channel blocker, Parkinson's disease, aplastic anemia
    C. Synthetic nucleoside analog, chronic hepatitis C, cardiac arrest
    D. HMG-CoA reductase inhibitor, hyperlipidemia, rhabdomyolysis

52. **Which of the following drugs is used to treat rheumatoid arthritis?**

    A. Tolcapone
    B. Etanercept
    C. Topiramate
    D. Risdronate.

53. Which of the following is not likely to be used in the treatment of iron deficiency anemia?

   A. Ferrous sulfate, PO
   B. Dextran 40, IV
   C. Sodium ferric gluconate, IV
   D. Iron sucrose, PO

54. Which of the following is FALSE concerning the use of NSAIDs for pain management?

   A. NSAIDs are analgesic and anti-inflammatory.
   B. NSAIDs inhibit prostaglandin synthesis via the lipo-oxygenase pathway.
   C. NSAIDs can cause GI upset and GI bleeds.
   D. Indomethacin should not be taken in excess of 200 mg per day.

55. What does the "B" in the chemotherapeutic combination, ABVD represent?

   A. Bleomycin
   B. Baclofen
   C. Bivalirudin
   D. Buspirone

56. Imuran is used as an immunosuppressant to prevent kidney transplant rejection. Which of the following should be monitored in a patient on Imuran?

I. Amylase and lipase levels
II. Liver Function Tests (LFTs)
III. CBC with differential
IV. Creatine phosphokinase levels

   A. I only
   B. II only
   C. I, II and III only
   D. IV only

57. Which of the following drugs is used to treat tuberculosis?

   A. Pyrazinamide
   B. Celecoxib
   C. Propoxyphene
   D. None of the above

58. For the following chemotherapeutic agents, determine the INCORRECT combination of agent/mechanism of action.

I. Olanzapine/ Dopamine and Serotonin-2 receptor antagonist
II. Paclitaxel/anti-mitotic
III. Pindolol/ beta-adrenergic antagonist
IV. Donepezil/alkylating agent

   A. I and II only
   B. II and IV only
   C. III and IV only
   D. IV only

59. **Which of the following are anti-arrhythmics?**

   A. Ondansetron
   B. Filgrastim
   C. Zolpidem
   D. None of the above

60. **Which of the following statements is true concerning Cholecalciferol?**

   A. It is contraindicated in hypercalcemia.
   B. One needs to monitor a patient on cholecalciferol for possible thromboembolic events.
   C. Statement B is true, but statement A is false.
   D. Both statements A and B are true.

61. **Which of the following would be useful as an effective anti-androgen therapy in a 78-year-old patient with prostate cancer?**

I. Bilateral orchiectomy.
II. A testosterone antagonist such as bicalutamide only.
III. An LH-RH antagonist such as cetrorelix.

   A. I only
   B. III only
   C. I and/or III
   D. II only

62. **What is the mechanism of action of mycophenolate mofetil (CellCept)?**

   A. Mycophenolate mofetil is a neurokinin-1 antagonist used to prevent chemotherapy-induced nausea and vomiting.
   B. Mycophenolate mofetil is a 5HT3 antagonist used to prevent post-operative nausea.
   C. Mycophenolate mofetil is a corticosteroid analog used as an immunosuppressant.
   D. Mycophenolate mofetil is an immunosuppressant used to prevent organ rejection.

63. **Of the following medications, which is the only neuromuscular blocker?**

   A. Botulinum toxin A
   B. Oxcabazepine
   C. Chlordiazepoxide
   D. Finasteride

64. **A 23-year-old female patient has been diagnosed with bipolar disorder. Which of the following would be the best therapeutic approach?**

   A. An antipsychotic such as aripiprazole
   B. An anxiolytic such as azothioprine.
   C. A calcium regulator such as zoledronic acid
   D. A mood stabilizer such as lithium or lamotrigine.

65. **Which of the following is NOT an atypical antipsychotic?**

    A. Quetiapine.
    B. Olanzapine
    C. Clozapin
    D. Amitriptyline

66. **Which of the following are TRUE sign/symptoms/complications of anemia of chronic kidney disease?**

I. Red blood cells are macrocytic and the MCV (mean corpuscular volume) is normal.
II. The hematocrit is low, usually less than 30.
III. The red blood cells are normocytic and normochromic.
IV. Fatigue, irritability, sore tongue, shortness of breath and weakness are all common symptoms.

    A. I and II only
    B. II and III only
    C. I, II, and III only
    D. II, III and IV only

67. **Which of the following is a brand name for irbesartan?**

    A. Nimotop
    B. Plendil
    C. Avapro
    D. Plaquenil

68. **You are preparing an insulin infusion. Which of the following should NOT be combined with insulin in an IV?**

    A. Heparin
    B. Hydrocortisone.
    C. Nitroglycerin
    D. Potassium chloride

69. **Which of the following would be considered a contraindication for the use of docusate?**

    A. Pregnancy
    B. Hip dysplasia
    C. IDDM
    D. Intestinal obstruction

70. **Which of the following drugs is an opioid agonist?**

    A. Dapsone
    B. Rifapentine
    C. Pyrazinamide
    D. Meperidine

71. **Why is carbidopa added to levodopa for the treatment of Parkinson's disease?**
    A. It prevents degradation of levodopa in the periphery.
    B. It minimizes some of the side effects of levodopa used alone.
    C. Addition of carbidopa stabilizes levodopa by interfering with Phase III metabolism.
    D. Carbidopa complexes with levodopa to allow increased solubility.

72. **Which of the following forms is methumazole available in?**

I. Troche
II. Tablet
III. Cream
IV. Capsule

    A. I only
    B. II only
    C. II and IV only
    D. Methimazole is available in all the listed forms.

73. **Which of the following is the generic name of Altace?**
    A. Zonisamide
    B. Lovastatin
    C. Lisinopril
    D. Ramipil

74. **Which of the following is potential side effect of lovastatin?**
    A. Pruritis, rash
    B. Hepatic necrosis/hepatotoxicity
    C. Myalgia, cramping
    D. All of the above

75. **Which of the following are possible adverse effects of methotrexate?**

I. Leukoencephalopathy
II. Tubular necrosis
III. Hepatotoxicity
IV. GI bleed

    A. I and II only
    B. II and III only
    C. I and III only
    D. All of the above are possible adverse effects.

76. **Which of the following medications is a Pregnancy Category X?**
    A. Rivastigmine
    B. Dronobinol
    C. Infliximab
    D. Methotrexate

77. **Which of the following tablets and capsules should NOT be crushed?**

I. Boniva
II. Inderide
III. OxyContin
IV. Propylthiouracil

    A. I only
    B. II only
    C. I, II and III only
    D. IV only

78. **Which of the following statement(s) about A1c is/are untrue?**

    A. Measurement of A1c correlates approximately with the lifespan of a red blood cell, about 6-8 months.
    B. Normal A1c should be at 4-6%.
    C. A1c gives an approximation of glucose control in a patient corresponding to the previous 3-4 months.
    D. A1c will also be raised in chronic renal failure.

79. **Which of the following is a loop diuretic?**

    A. Verapamil
    B. Adenosine
    C. Propafenone
    D. Bumetanide

80. **Which of the following are ACE inhibitors?**

I. Benzapril
II. Ramipril
III. Losartan

    A. All of the above
    B. None of the above
    C. I only
    D. I and II only

81. **Which of the following is an appropriate agent and dosing schedule for a newly diagnosed patient with gout?**

    A. Acarbose, 100mg, PO, tid
    B. Alitretinoin, 0.1% topical gel, qid
    C. Hydroxycobalamin, 500mcg, PO, qd
    D. Allopurinol, 200 mg PO, qd

82. **What do the "B" and the "M" in the chemotherapeutic combination BEAM represent?**

    A. BCNU (carmustine) and melphalan
    B. Bendamustine and melphalan
    C. BCNU (carmustine) and meloxicam
    D. Bleomycin and Matulane (procarbazine)

83. **Which of the following trade names is NOT correctly matched with its generic name?**

    A. Nitazoxanide-Alinia
    B. Nisoldipine-Sular
    C. Felopidine -Plendil
    D. Rifaximin-Zifaxanilimide

84. **What is the therapeutic class of itracozanole (Sporanox)?**

    A. Itracozanole is an anti-fungal agent.
    B. Itracozanole is an antibacterial agent.
    C. Itracozanole is an antiviral agent.
    D. Itracozanole is a GABA agonist.

85. **Which of the following is potential side effect of pindolol?**

I. Erectile dysfunction
II. Hypoglycemia
III. Bronchospasm
IV. Heart failure

    A. I and II only
    B. I and III only
    C. IV only
    D. All of the above

86. **Of the following medications, which is also known as phytonadione?**

    A. Vitamin A
    B. Vitamin E
    C. Vitamin D
    D. Vitamin K

87. **Which of the following is a calcium channel blocker?**

    A. Aripiprazole
    B. Modafinil
    C. Moricizine
    D. Nifedipine

88. **Repaglinide is a(n) _____ used to treat _____ and rarely has the adverse effect of inducing _____.**

    A. Non-selective beta-blocker, hypotension, tachycardia.
    B. Hypoglycemic, diabetes, hypoglycemia.
    C. Anti-psychotic, schizophrenia, psychotic breaks.
    D. Platelet inhibitor, post-MI, bleeding.

89. **Which of the following are signs/symptoms/complications of an adverse reaction to sulfisoxazole?**

    A. Diarrhea
    B. Shortness of breath, dyspnea
    C. Hypertension
    D. Both A and B are possible symptoms.

90. **Which of the following medications is a bisphosphonate?**
    A. Methotrexate
    B. Alendronate
    C. Ribavarin
    D. Orlistat

91. **Which of the following is a brand name for Orlistat?**
    A. Xenical
    B. Zenicote
    C. Xenibrium
    D. Xenlast

92. **Which of the following is a phosphodiesterase inhibitor?**
    A. Verapamil
    B. Furosemide
    C. Budenoside
    D. Sindenafil

93. **Which of the following drugs are removed during hemodialysis?**

I. Allopurinol
II. Metoprolol
III. Metformin
    A. I only
    B. II only
    C. I, II and III
    D. III only

94. **Which of the following drugs are removed during peritoneal dialysis?**

I. Carisopradol
II. Mannitol
III. Methyldopa
    A. I only
    B. II only
    C. I, II and III
    D. III only

95. **Which of the following would be considered a precaution for the use of inamrinone?**

I. Serious infection
II. Renal or hepatic disease
III. Valvular disease
IV. A history of depression
    A. I and II only
    B. II and III only
    C. I, II and III only
    D. All of the above

-19-

96. **Which of the following would be the most likely first line of therapy in a 38-year-old male with a bp of 140/78 and migraines?**
    A. Thiazide diuretic
    B. Calcium channel blockers or ACE inhibitors
    C. Angiotensin II receptor blockers or Na$^+$ channel blockers
    D. There is no prophylactic treatment for migraines

97. **To which class of drugs do following belong?**

I. Aminophylline
II. Salmetrol
III. Isoproterenol

    A. Antihypertensives
    B. Hypoglycemics
    C. Platelet inhibitors
    D. Bronchodilators

98. **Which of the following drugs are bronchodilators and used to treat asthma?**

I. Albuterol
II. Isoproterenol
III. Terbutaline
IV. Mirtazapine

    A. All of the above
    B. None of the above
    C. I, II and III only
    D. I and II only

99. **Which of the following forms is cyclosporine available in?**

I. IV injectable
II. Topical gel, cream, patch or spray
III. Capsule

    A. I only
    B. I and III only
    C. II only
    D. Cyclosporine is available in all the listed forms.

100. **To which class of anti-infectives does ofloxacin (Floxin, Ocuflox) belong?**

    A. 2nd generation cephalosporin
    B. Fluoroquinoline
    C. Sulfonamides
    D. Monobactam

101. **What is sumatriptan used to treat?**
    A. Grave's disease
    B. Acute migraine
    C. Hypothyroidism
    D. Adrenal fatigue

102. **Which of the following are possible adverse effects of sumatriptan (Imitrex)?**

I. Coronary vasospasm
II. Myocardial infarction
III. Hepatotoxicity

    A. I and II only
    B. II and III only.
    C. I and III only
    D. All of the above are possible adverse effects.

103. **Which of the following conditions is a contraindication for the use of danazol/Danocrine?**
    A. Pregnancy or lactation
    B. Anemia
    C. A history of diabetes
    D. A history of intestinal obstruction

104. **Which of the following are used to prevent and treat gout?**

I. NSAIDs
II. Colchicine
III. Corticosteroids
IV. Allopurinol

    A. I and II only
    B. II and III only
    C. II and IV only
    D. All of the above

105. **Which of the following is an appropriate agent and dosing schedule for managing obesity?**
    A. Orlistat, 120mg, PO, tid
    B. Lepirudin, 0.15/kg (IV)
    C. Lovastatin, 20mg, PO, qd
    D. Ranitidine, 50mg, IM, q 6-8 hrs.

106. **When discussing antibiotic treatment (penicillin G, 500 mg, PO, tid) with a patient, which of the following is true?**

I. There are no interactions to be concerned about with penicillin G.
II. If a patient is on oral contraceptives, it is strongly suggested that a backup means of contraception is used.
III. If a patient is on oral contraceptives, it is strongly suggested that they stop using the contraceptives immediately.
IV. Taking oral contraceptives along with penicillin is fine as long as you double up on the oral contraceptive.

    A. I only
    B. II only
    C. III only
    D. IV only

107. **A patient is in hypertensive crisis with bp> 240/130 mm Hg. There is evidence of end organ damage. Which of the following would be the BEST first choice to use?**

    A. Labetalol
    B. Hydralazine, IV
    C. Clonidine
    D. Nitroprusside, IV

108. **In the TNM staging system, what does the "N" stand for?**

    A. Degree of tumor differentiation
    B. Nodal involvement
    C. Tumor number
    D. Tumor type

109. **Of the following generic and brand names, which are INCORRECTLY matched?**

    A. Fluticasone, Flonase.
    B. Miglitol, Glyset
    C. Matinamab, Gleevec
    D. Pramipexole, Mirapex

110. **Which of the following is an angiotensin-converting enzyme inhibitor?**

    A. Aripiprazole.
    B. Univasc
    C. Piroxicam
    D. Edrophonium

111. **Which of the following forms is pyridostigmine available in?**

I. IM injectable
II. IV injectable
III. Tablet
IV. Syrup

    A. I only
    B. I, II and III only
    C. All of the above
    D. III and IV only

112. **Which of the following drugs are used to treat Parkinson's disease?**

I. Albuterol
II. Entacapone
III. Zoledronic acid
IV. Liotrix

    A. All of the above
    B. None of the above
    C. I, II and III only
    D. II only

113. **Tolbutamide is a(n) _____ used to treat _____ and rarely has the adverse effect of inducing _____.**

    A. Hypoglycemic, NIDDM, SIADH
    B. Anti-hypertensive, acute hypertensive crisis, atrial fibrillation
    C. Antidepressant, ADD, thrombocytopenia
    D. Dopamine antagonist, insomnia, thrombocytosis

114. **If a patient is on a potassium sparing diuretic, which of the following lab values should be monitored?**

    A. Electrolytes
    B. Serum glucose
    C. Blood pressure
    D. Both blood pressure and serum electrolytes should be monitored.

115. **Which of the following are vasodilators?**

I. Minoxidil
II. Isosorbide
III. Bosentan

    A. I and II only
    B. All of the above
    C. I only.
    D. II and III only

116. **Which of the following conditions is a contraindication/precaution for the use of immunosuppressants?**

I. Severe infection
II. Uncompensated heart failure
III. Pregnant patients with RA

    A. I only
    B. II only
    C. III only
    D. I, II and III

117. **Which of the following would be the BEST option for the treatment of psoriasis?**

    A. Basilixamab
    B. Topotecan
    C. Paclitaxel
    D. Topical corticosteroids

118. **A clinical trial is studying the response of 2 independent groups. If numeric scales are used, which of the following would be the preferred mode of statistical analysis?**

    A. ANOVA
    B. Paired t-tests
    C. Mann-Whitney
    D. Chi-square

119. **Which of the following drugs is NOT an antineoplastic?**

    A. Carmustine
    B. Alendronate
    C. Etoposide
    D. Gemcitabine

120. **Lexxel is a combination of which medications?**

    A. Emtricitabine, disoproxil
    B. Hydrocholorothiazide (HCTZ), Losartan
    C. Enalapril, felodipine
    D. Amylase, lipase and protease

121. **Which of the following is galantamine used to treat?**

I. Seizures
II. Myocarditis
III. Alzheimer's disease
IV. Mild cognitive dysfunction

    A. I only
    B. II only
    C. III only
    D. All of the above

122. **Which of the following are possible signs/symptoms/complications of respiratory alkalosis?**

I. Apathy
II. Confusion
III. Air hunger
IV. Muscle twitching

    A. II and III only
    B. II and IV only
    C. All of the above
    D. III only

123. **Which of the following are signs of agranulocytemia?**

I. Chills
II. Fever
III. Hallucinations

    A. I and II only
    B. II and III only
    C. I and III only
    D. All of the above are possible adverse effects.

124. **Which of the following statement(s) about venlafaxine is/are untrue?**

    A. Depression and generalized anxiety disorder are indications.
    B. MAOI use is contraindicated.
    C. It can be used to treat panic disorder.
    D. It is generally given as a weekly IM injection on an outpatient basis.

125. **Which of the following is NOT a normal lab value?**

    A. Cardiac troponin < 1mcg/mL
    B. Prostate Specific Antigen (PSA) > 50 ng/mL
    C. Glucose: 70-100 mg/mL
    D. Hemoglobin:15 g/dL

126. **Which of the following are not useful in the treatment of hypertension?**

I. Enalapril
II. Lisinopril
III. Alfentanil

    A. All of the above
    B. None of the above
    C. III only
    D. I and II only

127. **Which of the following would be used for SLOW induction of anesthesia and for maintenance?**

    A. Ropivicaine
    B. Pancuronium
    C. Thiopental
    D. Fentenyl

128. **Which of the following drugs is a combination product used for pain relief?**

    A. Atamet
    B. Endocet
    C. Epzicom
    D. Zestoretic

129. **What is the mechanism of action of irbesartan (Avapro)?**

    A. Irbesartan is an anti-cholinergic agent.
    B. Irbesartan is a norepinephrine / serotonin reuptake inhibitor.
    C. Irbesartan is an angiotensin II receptor antagonist.
    D. Irbesartan is a GABA agonist.

130. **Of the following medications, which is the only hypoglycemic agent?**

    A. Paroxetine
    B. Nateglinide
    C. Tocainide
    D. Magnesium oxide

131. **Of the following lab values, which show correct normal values?**

I. WBC, 4000-11,000/mm3
II. Cardiac troponin I < 10mcg/mL
III. TSH 0.5-4.8 mIU/mL
IV. Fasting glucose: 70-100 mg/dL.

    A. I only
    B. I and II only
    C. I and III only
    D. All of the above

132. **For which of the following infusion rates is the mass of the patient important?**

I. Dopamine
II. Phenylephrine
III. Epinephrine
IV. Nitroglycerin

    A. I and II only
    B. I, II and III only
    C. I only
    D. IV only

133. **Which of the following drugs is a large, dark blue tablet?**
    A. Valtrex, 1000 mg
    B. Venlafaxine, 100mg
    C. Zocor, 80 mg
    D. Amoxicillin, 875 mg

134. **Olanzapine is a(n) _____ used to treat _____ and rarely has the adverse effect of inducing _____.**
    A. Anti-psychotic, schizophrenia, neuroleptic malignant syndrome
    B. Antidepressant, seasonal affective disorder, bradycardia
    C. Antiepileptic, partial seizures, agranulocytosis
    D. Serotonin agonist, nausea and vomiting of pregnancy, spontaneous abortion

135. **Which of the following are NOT signs/symptoms of anaphylaxis?**
    A. Urticaria
    B. Wheezing
    C. Angioedema
    D. Dyspnea

136. **Which is the supplement that contains a natural statin?**
    A. Shark cartilage
    B. Red Yeast Rice
    C. Saw palmetto
    D. Echinacea

137. **Which of the following medications is a neuromuscular blocker?**
    A. Milrinone
    B. Amlodipine
    C. Finasteride
    D. Vecuronium

138. **Which of the following is a brand name for olanzapine?**
    A. Zyprexa, Zydis
    B. Lanza
    C. Quiettime
    D. Prozac

139. **Leucovorin can be given as a "rescue therapy" for which of the following?**
    A. Doxorubicin
    B. Methotrexate
    C. Cytarabine
    D. None of the above

140. **A patient is newly diagnosed with folic acid deficiency and megaloblastic anemia. What is the appropriate dosage for a child older than 4 years old?**

    A. 400 mcg qd, IV, IM or sc
    B. 5 mg/mL bid, IV or sc
    C. 30 mg qd, PO only
    D. 300 mg, qd, PO only

141. **Which of the following forms is tamoxifen available in?**

I. IM injectable
II. IV injectable
III. Tablets
IV. Oral solution

    A. I only
    B. I, II and III only
    C. III and IV only
    D. All the listed forms are available.

142. **Which of the following is the brand name of hydroxyquinolone?**

    A. Plaquenil
    B. Quinapril
    C. Quinate
    D. Quixin

143. **What is prazosin used to treat?**

    A. Grave's disease.
    B. Hypertension
    C. Hypercholesterolemia
    D. Homocyteinemia

144. **Which of the following are possible adverse effects of tenecteplase (TNKase)?**

I. Intracranial hemorrhage
II. Cardiovascular events
III. Constipation

    A. I and II only
    B. II and III only
    C. I and III only
    D. All of the above are possible adverse effects.

145. **Which of the following is the presumed action of saw palmetto?**

    A. Treatment of BPH by inhibition of 5-α-reductase
    B. Prevention of colds by an immune-stimulatory action
    C. Treatment of hypercholesterolemia by inhibition of HMG-CoA-reductase
    D. Treatment of hypercoagulable states by the inhibition of platelet adhesion

146. **Which of the following are some of the most commonly prescribed drugs?**

I. Lortab/hydrocodone
II. Zoloft/sertraline
III. Leukine/sargramostim

    A. I and II only
    B. All of the above
    C. I only.
    D. II and III only.

147. **Which of the following is an appropriate diagnosis for the use of Gleevec?**

    A. Transplant rejection
    B. Oat cell carcinoma
    C. Chronic myelogenous leukemia (CML)
    D. Acute migraine

148. **To what class of drugs does ketoprofen belong?**

    A. NSAID
    B. Biological response modifiers
    C. Antipsychotic
    D. Alkylating agents

149. **Which of the following is another term for Vitamin B_{12}?**

    A. Phytonadione
    B. Cyanocobalamin
    C. Cholecalciferol
    D. Pyridoxine

150. **Which of the following drugs should NOT be used as a diuretic?**

I. Albuterol
II. Acetazolamide
III. Mannitol
IV. Metolazone

    A. All of the above
    B. I only
    C. II, III and IV only
    D. I and II only

151. **Tramadol is a(n) _____ used to treat _____ and rarely has the adverse effect of inducing _____.**

    A. Thiazide diuretic, ascites, electrolyte imbalance
    B. Anti-infective, penicillin derivative, community acquired pneumonia, thrombocytopenia
    C. Atypical antipsychotic, bipolar disorder, acute manic episodes
    D. Opioid agonist, moderate to severe pain, respiratory depression

152. **Which of the following are possible signs/symptoms/complications of tretinoin (Retin-A)?**

I. GI hemorrhage.
II. Cerebrovascular accident
III. Disseminated intravascular coagulation (DIC)

    A. All of the above
    B. None of the above
    C. I only
    D. I and III only

153. **Which of the following physiological processes does grapefruit juice interfere with?**

    A. Phase I liver metabolism
    B. Kreb's Cycle
    C. Electron transport chain
    D. All of the above

154. **If a patient is on Lanoxin, what is the likely diagnosis?**

    A. Urinary tract infection
    B. Heart failure
    C. Hypertension
    D. Stevens-Johnson syndrome

155. **Which of the following are potential interactions with duloxetine/Cymbalta?**

    A. Alcohol use increases risk of hepatic damage.
    B. Use along with warfarin increases risk of GI bleed.
    C. Both A and B
    D. Neither A nor B

156. **Which of the following is an anti-retroviral agent?**

    A. Acyclovir
    B. Indinavir
    C. Famcyclovir
    D. Valaciclovir

157. **Vytorin is a combination of which two medications?**

    A. Miconazole with $NaHCO_3$
    B. Carbidopa and levodopa
    C. HCTZ and propranol
    D. Ezetimide and simvastatin

158. **Which of the following is a potential serious side effect of Zyrtec-D?**

    A. Bronchospasm
    B. Dysphagia
    C. Diarrhea
    D. Pruritis

159. **What is dalteparin/Fragmin used to treat?**

   A. Essential hypertension
   B. Deep vein thromboses
   C. Constipation
   D. Viral infections.

160. **Which of the following is potential side effect of phenazopyridine (Prodium, Pyridiate, Urogesic)?**

I. Renal toxicity
II. Hemolytic anemia
III. Hepatotoxicity
IV. Bright orange urine

   A. I only
   B. II only
   C. III only
   D. All of the above

161. **What might nizatidine (Axid) be prescribed for?**

I. Situational depression
II. Active duodenal ulcer
III. Mild seasonal affective disorder (SAD)
IV. Gastroesophageal reflux disease (GERD)

   A. I and III only
   B. II and IV only
   C. All of the above
   D. None of the above

162. **Which of the following medications comes as a capsule?**

   A. Lotrel
   B. Norvasc
   C. Xanax
   D. Fosamax

163. **Which of the following drugs are metabolized via the CYP3A4 pathway?**

   A. Warfarin
   B. Alprazolam
   C. Theophylline
   D. Fluoxetine

164. **A patient is considering switching from Catapres patch to the Catapres tablet. Which of the following is the best suggestion you would give them?**

   A. Never use both the patch and the tablets together.
   B. Use both the patch and the tablets for 2-3 days before stopping the patch.
   C. Leave the patch off for 5-7 days and then begin using the tablets.
   D. None of the above; the Catapres patch is ineffective.

165. **Which of the following should NOT be used to prevent a migraine?**

   A. OTC products with caffeine
   B. Anti-depressants
   C. Anti-hypertensives
   D. OTC migraine analgesics

166. **Which of the following is given for post-operative nausea and vomiting?**

   A. Dolora
   B. Actiq
   C. Droperidol
   D. Fentora

167. **Which of the following forms is phenobarbital available in?**

I. Elixir: 20mg/5 mL
II. Pre-filled syringes (50 mg/mL in 2 mL syringes)
III. Suppositories (30, 120, 200 mg)
IV. Capsule: 100 mg
V. Tablets, timed release (100, 200 mg)

   A. II and V only
   B. I, II, III and IV only
   C. III only
   D. III and IV only

168. **Which of the following drugs is an anti-platelet agent?**

   A. Inamrinone
   B. Benzotropine
   C. Busulfan
   D. Clopidogrel

169. **Which of the following makes an incorrect statement concerning the administration of Cholestyramine?**

   A. Take the medicine with any carbonated beverage because it increases absorption.
   B. Take the medicine with water only.
   C. You can take the medicine with either water or food.
   D. Answers B and C are correct

170. **Which of the following class of drugs is used as anti-emetics?**

   A. Fluroquinolones
   B. MAO Inhibitors
   C. 5HT-3 receptor antagonists
   D. HMG-CoA reductase inhibitors.

171. **Which of the following drugs is a hypoglycemic?**

   A. Glipizide
   B. Sirolimus
   C. Tiotropium
   D. Olmesartan

172. **A 28-year-old female patient is diagnosed with Graves' disease. She is placed on liothyronine. Why is that inappropriate?**

   A. Liothyronine is synthetic T3. Graves' disease is a state of hyperthyroidism, and Liothyronine is contraindicated..
   B. It is not inappropriate; use of liothyronine follows current practice guidelines.
   C. She should be given Levothyroxine instead; the Levothyroxine will be converted *in vivo* to T3.
   D. Liothyronine is a Category X drug and should not be given to females of child bearing age.

173. **Which of the following drugs is contraindicated for a 28-year-old female taking oral contraceptives?**

I. Macrolides
II. Rotinavir
III. Barbiturates

   A. I only
   B. II only
   C. III only
   D. All of the above

174. **Which of the following drugs is an angiotensin II receptor antagonist?**

   A. Glipizide
   B. Olmesartan
   C. Repaglinide
   D. Sirolimus

175. **A patient is diagnosed and cholestyramine is prescribed. What is the likely diagnosis?**

   A. Hypertension
   B. Herpes simplex infection
   C. Type 2 diabetes
   D. Biliary obstruction

176. **Of the following methods of administration, which is the best advice for a patient taking a bisphosphonate?**

   A. Take with as small amount of food or water as possible.
   B. Take in the morning at least 30 minutes before any meal. Drink a full glass of water with the bisphosphonate.
   C. Take anytime during the day when convenient.
   D. Bisphosphonates should be taken at night to minimize gastric upset.

177. **Of the following drugs, which is an anticonvulsant?**

I. Carbamazepine
II. Fondaparinux
III. Lamotrigine

    A. I only
    B. II only
    C. III only
    D. I and III only

178. **In which of the following is the brand name for an inhalation form of insulin?**

    A. Exubera
    B. Humulin
    C. NovoLog
    D. Lantus

179. **Which of the following drugs is a platelet aggregation inhibitor?**

    A. Pyrazinamide
    B. Etanercept
    C. Ticlodipine
    D. Ziprasidone

180. **A patient using moricizine (Ethmozine) approaches you asking what possible side effects there might be. What could you tell him?**

I. Arrhythmias
II. Thrombophlebitis
III. Pseudomembranous colitis

    A. I only
    B. II only
    C. I and II only
    D. All are possible side effects.

181. **Which of the following drugs is an MAOI (monoamine oxidase inhibitor)?**

    A. Selegiline
    B. Sotalol
    C. Trazodone
    D. Sorafenib

182. **A 42-year-old female is on moricizine, 600mg PO, qd. Which of the following tests would be MOST vital to follow?**

I. ECGs
II. Fluid balance
III. Blood pressure levels
IV. Bowel movements

- A. I only
- B. I and II only
- C. I, II and III only
- D. II and IV only.

183. **Which of the following drugs is a calcium channel blocker?**

- A. Bethanechol
- B. Amlodipine
- C. Benzapril
- D. Alfentanil

184. **Which of the following is a brand name for Monteleukast?**

- A. MontKast
- B. SingKast
- C. Sinkumont
- D. Singulair

185. **Which of the following is a long-acting insulin?**

- A. Humulin50/50
- B. Humalog
- C. Novolog
- D. Ultralente

186. **What are the drugs combined in Maxzide, and what is the indication?**

- A. Amiloride, HCTZ, diuresis
- B. HCTZ, triamterene, cardiac arrythmias
- C. HCTZ, triamterene, hypertension
- D. Guaifenisin, theophylline, asthma

187. **Which of the following disorders is a contraindication for the use of naratriptan?**

- A. Basilar headaches
- B. Acne vulgaris
- C. A history of breast cancer
- D. SLE

188. **Which of the following is used to treat psoriasis?**

- A. Vitamin K analogs
- B. Vitamin D analogs
- C. Vitamin A analogs
- D. Vitamin E analogs

189. **Which is the correct conversion from grams to grains?**

    A. 1 gram =15.43 grains
    B. 1 gram = 60 grains
    C. 1 gram = 1 minim
    D. 1 gram = 1 fluid ounce

190. **Which of the following conditions would indicate a need for caution in a patient on psuedophedrine?**

I. Sinus headaches
II. Hyperthyroidism
III. Glaucoma
IV. Concurrent viral infections

    A. I and II only
    B. II and III only
    C. II and IV only
    D. None of the above require caution

191. **You are given an order that reads: Tamoxifen 200 mg PO bid. What should be your next step?**

    A. Call the prescribing physician with a question about the dose.
    B. Dispense as prescribed.
    C. Dispense as prescribed, but note your concerns on the record.
    D. Call the prescribing physician with a question about the route of delivery.

192. **A 28-year-old female patient has just started taking Xanax and is concerned that it may not be safe if she decides to try and get pregnant. Which of the following adverse effects would not be mentioned during your counseling session with her?**

    A. Blood dyscrasias
    B. Xanax is a Pregnancy Category D drug.
    C. Seizures may accompany abrupt withdrawal.
    D. Hyperkalemia, hyponatremia

193. **Which of the following drugs could be used as a decongestant in a 6-year-old child?**

    A. Pseudophedrine
    B. Psyllium
    C. Sirolimus
    D. Sulfisoxazole

194. **Which of the following has a "black box warning" associated with it?**

I. Celecoxib
II. Ibuprofen
III. ACE inhibitors
IV. Acarbose

    A. I only
    B. I and II only
    C. I, II and III only
    D. All of the above

195. **You are seeing an elderly patient with congestive heart failure. Both nesiritide and bosentan have been recommended for this patient. Which of the following statements are true, if any?**

    A. Nesiritide should not be used in patients with a systolic pressure under 90mm Hg. Bosentan may be used in these patients.
    B. Bosentan is an ACE inhibitor and should be used cautiously in elderlypatients with pulmonary hypertension.
    C. Both A and B are correct.
    D. A is correct, but B is incorrect. The systolic pressure may safely be less than 90mm Hg as long as the patient is continuously monitored.

196. **Which of the following is a NOT a disease-modifying agent used to treat RA?**

    A. Azothiaprine
    B. Minoxidil
    C. Methotrexate
    D. Auranofin

197. **Which of the following drugs are CYP2D6 inhibitors?**

I. Amiodorone/Cirdarone
II. Imatamib/Gleevec
III. Thioridazine/Mellaril
IV. Terbinafine/Lamisil

    A. I and II only
    B. I, II and III only
    C. II only
    D. All of the above

198. **A patient with a diagnosis of myasthenia gravis has a prescription for Prostigmin. In what forms is Prostigmin available?**

I. Prostigmin is available as 2, 1, 0.5 and 0.25 mg/mL injections.
II. Prostigmin is available as 15 mg tablets.
III. Prostigmin is available only as an injection, and the patient must be trained in self-administration.
IV. Prostigmin is available as both injection and tablet forms, and atropine should be readily available to treat possible cholinergic crises.

    A. I only
    B. II only
    C. I and III only
    D. IV

199. **A patient diagnosed with Type II Diabetes asks you to explain how to take her medication. The prescription is for Glucotrol (glypizide) 20 mg/day. Glucotrol comes in 10mg extended-release tablets. The label reads: Take two tablets 3 times a day after mealtime by dissolving under the tongue. What is/are the error(s) on the label?**

    A. The tablet should be swallowed and not dissolved under the tongue.
    B. Two 10mg tablets should be taken before breakfast, not three times a day, and not after a meal, but ~30minutes before a meal.
    C. The tablet should be taken after meals on a full stomach.
    D. Both A and B are correct.

200. **Which is the correct conversion from drahms to ounces?**

    A. 8 drahm = 1 fluid ounce
    B. 1 drahm = 8 fluid ounces
    C. 1 drahm = 60 fluid ounces
    D. 8 drahm = 60 fluid ounces

201. **Which is the correct conversion from teaspoons to drahms?**

    A. 8 teaspoons = 1 drahm
    B. 1.3 teaspoons = 1 drahm
    C. 1 teaspoon = 1.3 drahm
    D. 8 teaspoons = 60 drahm

202. **Which of the following vitamins are water-soluble and are excreted in the urine?**

I. Vitamin C
II. Vitamin B12
III. Vitamin A
IV. Beta-carotenes

    A. I and II only
    B. I and III only
    C. III and IV only
    D. I, II and IV only

203. **How many times should the label be read before administration?**
   A. Once
   B. At least twice
   C. Three times, at a minimum
   D. Oral orders are always sufficient.

204. **Which of the following is an anti-convulsant?**
   A. Celebrex
   B. Celexa
   C. Cerebyx
   D. None of the above are anti-convulsants.

205. **Which of the following is an anti-hypertensive?**
   A. Clonidine
   B. Norpramin
   C. Klonopin
   D. None of the above is an anti-hypertensive.

206. **Which of the following is an anti-psychotic?**
   A. Zyvox
   B. Zyrtec
   C. Zyprexa
   D. None of the above is an anti-psychotic.

207. **What are the most serious adverse effects of clindamycin?**

I. Pseudomembranous colitis
II. Neutropenia
III. Hepatic dysfunction

   A. I only
   B. II only
   C. III only
   D. I, II and III are all potential serious adverse effects.

208. **Which of the following abbreviations is no longer recommended for use due to potential medication errors?**
   A. qd
   B. PO
   C. iv
   D. im

209. **Which of the following methods of writing 100 micrograms is recommended for use to avoid potential medication errors?**
   A. .1mg
   B. 0.1mg
   C. 1/10 mg
   D. All are acceptable.

210. **Which of the following is an equivalent method of hand-writing 500 micrograms in a prescription or other record of medication?**

   A. 500 µg
   B. 500 mcg
   C. .5 mcg
   D. All are acceptable.

211. **Which of the following is an anti-protozoal agent?**

   A. Metronidazole
   B. Metformin
   C. Metoprolol
   D. Metolzone

212. **Which of the following should NOT be suggested for a patient on a prescription for tetracycline?**

   A. Avoid sunlight.
   B. Take with milk to avoid stomach upset.
   C. Do not use any alcohol while on tetracycline.
   D. Take oral form with at least 8 ounces of water 1 hour before a meal or 2 hours after eating a meal.

213. **A patient is taking 40 mg PO of lovastatin with his evening meal. He comes to you saying that for the last 2-3 weeks, he feels as if his legs are cramping. Which of the following tests would you recommended?**

   A. A CBC (complete blood count) and a full comp metabolic (chemistries) test
   B. Lipid levels including VLDL levels
   C. Total lovastatin serum concentrations
   D. Creatine phosphokinase (CPK), the MM isoenzyme

214. **Which of the following abbreviations is INCORRECTLY matched?**

   A. PO = per os (by mouth)
   B. tid = ter in die (3 times a day)
   C. qid = quater in die (once a day)
   D. All are correct.

215. **Which is the correct conversion from minims to milliliters (mL)?**

   A. 8 minims = 1 mL
   B. 1 minim = 15mL
   C. 15 minims = 1 mL
   D. 8 minims = 60 mL

216. **Of the following drugs, which are considered anti-hyperuricemic agents?**

I. Probenecid
II. Allopurinol
III. Dobutamine

    A. I and II only
    B. I and III only
    C. II and III only
    D. None of the three listed agents are anti-hyperuricemic agents.

217. **A patient using entecavir approaches you asking what possible side effects there might be. What could you tell him?**

I. HBV exacerbations
II. Lactic acidosis
III. Hepatomegaly

    A. I only
    B. II only
    C. II and III only
    D. All are possible side effects.

218. **Which of the following medications would be appropriate to treat a *Moraxella catarrhalis* infection in a child of 12 years?**

    A. Azithromycin
    B. Fluconozole
    C. Ampicillin
    D. Amoxicillin

219. **Of the following organisms, which would be susceptible to clindamycin?**

I. Staphyloccus
II. Bacteroides
III. Pseudomonas

    A. I and II only
    B. I, II and III only
    C. I and III only
    D. I only

220. **For which of the following conditions would QVAR be indicated?**

I. Seasonal/perennial rhinitis
II. Asthma
III. Emphysema

    A. I only
    B. II only
    C. III only
    D. I and II only

221. **Which of the following is used to measure forced vital capacity?**

   A. Spirometer
   B. Goniometer
   C. Sphygmomanometer
   D. Nebulizer

222. **Which of the following are common anti-emetics used as adjuncts in chemotherapy?**

I. Aprepitant
II. Ondansetron
III. Metoclopramide
IV. Palonosetron.

   A. I and III only
   B. II and IV only
   C. II and III only
   D. All are anti-emetics

223. **Which of the following is used to measure blood pressure?**

   A. Caliper
   B. Sphygmomanometer
   C. Spirometer
   D. Grave's speculum

224. **Loperimide is used to treat _____ and is contraindicated with/in _____.**

   A. Infection with Gram-negative bacteria, blood dyscrasias
   B. Osteomyelitis, severe hepatic disorders
   C. Diarrhea, acute diarrhea caused by *E coli*, *Salmonella* or *Shigella*
   D. Osteoporosis, leukemia

225. **Glipizide is a(n)_____ of the _____ class and is used to treat _____. Glipizide is contraindicated with/in _____.**

   A. Hypoglycemic, sulfonylurea, Type 2 diabetes, diabetic ketoacidosis (DKA)
   B. Hypoglycemic, biguanide, Type 1 diabetes, serious infection
   C. Hypoglycemic, thiozolidinedione, reactive hypoglycemia, children
   D. Anti-lipid agent, statin, hyperlipidemia, gout exacerbations

226. **Pioglitazone is a(n)_____ of the _____ class and is used to treat _____. Pioglitazone is contraindicated with/in _____.**

   A. Hypoglycemic, sulfonylurea, Type 2 diabetes, diabetic ketoacidosis (DKA)
   B. Hypoglycemic, biguanide, Type 1 diabetes, serious infection
   C. Hypoglycemic, thiozolidinedione, Type 2 diabetes, children.
   D. Anti-lipid agent, statin, hyperlipidemia, gout exacerbations

227. **You are working in a university hospital setting where many patients are enrolled in clinical trials. Which of the following statements is true concerning Phase I, II or III clinical trials?**

    A. A phase I trial is often very small (N<30) and seeks to determine the safe dose range for a new drug.
    B. A phase II trial is often larger than a phase I trial and seeks to determine if a new drug is effective enough to test in a phase III trial and to delineate adverse effects.
    C. A Phase III trial compares a new treatment with an established treatment and is usually much larger than either a phase I or a phase II trial.
    D. All three of the statements are correct.

228. **A patient diagnosed with PCOS (polycystic ovarian syndrome) is prescribed spironolactone along with a combined estrogen-progestin. What would you tell her about the serious possible side effects of the spironolactone?**

    A. The serious possible side effects include breast discomfort and increased urinary frequency.
    B. The serious possible side effects include breast discomfort and increased appetite.
    C. The serious possible side effects include GI bleeds, breast cancer, metaolic acidosis and hyperkalemia.
    D. The serious possible side effects include breast discomfort and increased breast size.

229. **A patient has an implanted coronary stent, and ticlopidine has been prescribed. Which of the following choices best complete the statement:**
Ticlopidine is a(n) _____. Major adverse reactions involve _____ and _____. _____ should NOT be taken concurrently with ticlopidine.

    A. Glycoprotein-receptor inhibitor, spinal hemorrhage, pulmonary hemorrhage, warfarin
    B. Platelet aggregation inhibitor, bleeding, bone marrow depression, aspirin
    C. Anti-coagulant, hemorrhage, hepatitis, hormonal contraceptives
    D. Vitamin-K inhibitor, uncontrolled bleeding, fever, aspirin

230. **Of the following medications, which is the only one used to treat asthma?**

    A. Androstenedione
    B. Zafirlukast
    C. Cytomel
    D. Finasteride

231. **A woman you have seen after the birth of her first child comes to you and tells you she has an at-home glucometer and regularly tests her blood sugar. It is sometimes a fasting blood sugar and sometimes not, but she remembers at least twice when she hadn't eaten for hours, her numbers were 148 and 160 mg/dL. What should you talk to her about?**

    A. Nothing; she doesn't have a blood glucose problem, but she probably should cut back on her sweets.
    B. She probably has insulin resistance, but it's not very serious yet. She should come back in a few months with more glucose readings.
    C. She probably is prediabetic, but can take her time getting any information.
    D. She has diabetes and would benefit from a professional diagnosis and formal classes on living with diabetes.

232. **Which of the following drugs is used to treat nausea and vomiting?**

    A. Tolcapone
    B. Butorphenol
    C. Topiramate
    D. Granisetron

233. **Which of the following are NOT typical symptoms/complications of serotonin syndrome?**

    A. Fever/chills with tremors
    B. Myoclonus, muscle rigidity, hyperreflexia
    C. Diaphoresis, agitation
    D. Headaches, diarrhea, anorexia

234. **Regarding pain management, which of the following statements is/are true of NSAIDs?**

I. NSAIDs are analgesic and anti-inflammatory.
II. Indomethacin should not be taken in excess of 200 mg per day.
III. NSAIDs can cause GI upset and GI bleeds.
IV. They inhibit prostaglandin synthesis via the cyclo-oxygenase pathway.

    A. All the statements are true.
    B. None of the statements are true.
    C. Statements I, II and IV are true.
    D. Statements I, II and III are true.

235. **A patient is diagnosed with an *H. pylori* associated ulcer. Which is generally the first-line treatment with such an ulcer?**

    A. OTC NSAIDs
    B. Antibiotics alone
    C. A proton pump inhibitor (PPI) plus antibiotics
    D. A proton pump inhibitor alone

236. **Which of the following is the brand name for hydrocortisone?**

I. Remicade
II. Cortef
III. Locoid
IV. Westcort

    A. I and II only
    B. II and IV only
    C. II, III and IV only
    D. I and IV only

237. **Inflixamab is used as an anti-imflammtory agent in rheumatoid arthritis (RA) and IBDs such as ulcerative colitis (UC) and Crohn's disease (CD). Which of the following should be monitored in a patient on inflixamab?**

I. Opportunistic infections
II. WBC and Platelet counts
III. Signs and symptoms of hypersensitivity including fever, chills, rash, dyspnea, facial flushing, chest pain and severe headache
IV. Creatine phosphokinase levels

    A. I only
    B. II only
    C. I, II and III only
    D. IV only

238. **Which of the following disorders is a contraindication for the use of moxifloxacin?**

    A. A history of systemic lupus erythematosis (SLE)
    B. A history of breast cancer
    C. A history of familial polyposis
    D. G6PD (glucose-6-phosphate dehydrogenase) deficiency

239. **What does the "R" in the chemotherapeutic combination, CHOP+R, represent?**

    A. Rituxan
    B. Ramelteon
    C. Ramipril
    D. Raloxiphene

240. **Which of the following is considered the "drug of choice" for *Clostridium difficile*?**

    A. Metronidazole
    B. Clindamycin
    C. Ketoconazole
    D. Ciprofloxacin

241. **What does the "D" in the chemotherapeutic combination, DICE, represent?**

    A. Denileukin
    B. Desipramine
    C. Diazepam
    D. Dexamethasone

242. **A patient has a glucose-6-phosphate dehydrogenase (G6PD) deficiency. Of the following drugs, which should be avoided in this patient?**

I. Quinolones
II. NSAIDs
III. Food colorings
IV. Vitamin B12

    A. I only
    B. II only
    C. I, II and III only
    D. All should be avoided

243. **For the following chemotherapeutic agents, determine the INCORRECT combination of agent and mechanism of action.**

I. Cyclophosphamide, alkylating agent
II. Paclitaxel, anti-mitotic
III. Leuprolide, gonadotropin-releasing hormone (GnRH) analog
IV. Procarbazine, alkylating agent

    A. I and II only
    B. II and IV only
    C. I, III and IV only
    D. All are correctly paired.

244. **Which of the following is/are NOT true of HIPAA (Health Insurance Portability and Accountability Act)?**

I. HIPAA does not address privacy issues.
II. One purpose was to improve the Medicare and Medicaid programs.
III. It is enforced by the Justice Department.
IV. HIPAA regulations apply to electronic healthcare transactions.

    A. Only I is not true.
    B. Both I and III are not true.
    C. All are true statements.
    D. Only IV is not a true statement.

245. **Brompheniramine is a _____ used to treat _____ and rarely has the adverse effect of inducing _____.**

    A. Histamine agonist, allergic rhinitis, hemolytic anemias
    B. Histamine-receptor agonist, anaphylaxis, aplastic anemia
    C. Anti-histamine, allergic symptoms, arrhythmias and bradycardia
    D. Epinephrin agonist, allergic symptoms, tachycardia

246. **Which of the following can induce a photoreaction in a sensitive individual?**

I. Diazepam
II. Naproxen
III. Nateglinide
IV. Vinblastine

    A. I and III only
    B. II and IV only
    C. I, II and III only
    D. III only

247. **Cytarabine is a nucleoside analog often used as a chemotherapeutic agent. Which of the following is true of chemically induced arachnoiditis on intrathecal injection?**

    A. Chemically induced arachnoiditis does not occur with cytarabine use.
    B. Dexamethasone should be co-administered to reduce arachnoiditis.
    C. Chemically induced arachnoiditis only occurs if the cytarabine is given too slowly. Otherwise, it is not a problem.
    D. An OTC analgesic should be co-administered with the cytarabine to limit chemically induced arachnoiditis.

248. **N-acetylcysteine is a(n) _____ used to treat _____ and is used as an antidote to _____ overdose.**

    A. Mucolytic, bronchitis, acetaminophen
    B. Voltage-gated Na channel blocker, hypertension, aplastic anemia
    C. Opioid antagonist, opiate withdrawal symptoms, heroin
    D. Serotonin antagonist, nausea and vomiting, Celecoxib

249. **Which of the following is a proton pump inhibitor (PPI)?**

    A. Ondansetron
    B. Filgrastim
    C. Atovastatin
    D. Pantoprazole

250. **Which of the following statements is true concerning SERMs (selective estrogen receptor modulators)?**

I. When using a SERM like tamoxifen, bone pain may be indicative of a good therapeutic response.
II. Individuals on SERMs may experience hot flashes.
III. Patients on SERMs must be monitored for possible thromboembolic events.
IV. At this point, it appears that all SERMs reduce the risk of breast cancer.

    A. I only
    B. I and II only
    C. II and IV only
    D. All are true statments.

251. **Which of the following would be an effective anti-androgen therapy in a 68-year-old patient with Stage II prostate cancer?**

I. Bilateral orchiectomy
II. A testosterone antagonist such as bicalutamide only
III. An LH-RH antagonist such as cetrorelix

   A. I only
   B. III only
   C. I and III
   D. II only

252. **What is the mechanism of action of fenofibrate (Tricor)?**

   A. Fenofibrate is a neurokinin-1 antagonist and an anti-emetic.
   B. Fenofibrate is a fibric acid derivative and an anti-hyperlipidemic agent.
   C. Fenofibrate is a corticosteroid analog and an immunosuppressant.
   D. Fenofibrate is a dopamine-2 agonist used to treat Parkinson's disease.

253. **Of the following medications, which is the only anxiolytic?**

   A. Doxepin
   B. Entacapone
   C. Alprazolam
   D. Finasteride

254. **Which of the following is an atypical antipsychotic?**

   A. Guaifenesin
   B. Haloperidol
   C. Temazepam
   D. Clozapine

255. **Which of the following drugs is an antipsychotic?**

   A. Dapsone
   B. Rifapentine
   C. Pyrazinamide
   D. Aripiprazole

256. **Which of the following drugs is used to treat osteoarthritis?**

I. Diclofenac
II. Celecoxib
III. Propoxyphene
IV. Guanfacine

   A. I, II and IV only
   B. II and IV only
   C. I, II and III only
   D. All the drugs listed are used to treat osteoarthritis.

257. **Acetoazolamide is a(n) _____ used to treat _____ and is contraindicated in _____.**

   A. Dopamine agonist, Parkinson's disease, hepatitis
   B. Carbonic anhydrase inhibitor, open-angle glaucoma and drug-induced edema, closed-angle glaucoma
   C. COX-2 inhibitor, osteoarthritis, chronic anemia
   D. Platelet aggregation inhibitor, atherosclerosis, high blood pressure

258. **Which of the following medications is a Pregnancy Category X?**

I. Methotrexate
II. Metronidazole
III. Atorvastatin
IV. Loratadine

   A. I only
   B. I and II only
   C. I, II and IV only
   D. I, II and III only

259. **Which of the following is the brand name of Zolpidem?**

   A. Ambien
   B. Modafinil
   C. Misoprostol
   D. Lisinopril

260. **When discussing contraception with a patient, which of the following is true?**

I. The use of either NuvaRing or Seasonale will not protect against Sexually Transmitted Infections (STIs)
II. A Seasonale user will likely have a period every three months
III. A NuvaRing should be inserted every three months

   A. I only.
   B. III only.
   C. I, II and III.
   D. I and II only

261. **Miglitol is a(n) _____ and a(n) _____ used to treat _____ and is contraindicated in _____.**

   A. Alpha-adrenergic blocker, antihypertensive, hypertension, cerebral edema
   B. Hypoglycemic agent, alpha-glucosidease inhibitor, Type 1 Diabetes, Type 2 diabetes
   C. Hypoglycemic agent, alpha-glucosidease inhibitor, Type 2 Diabetes, Type I diabetes
   D. Anti-coagulant, Vitamin K inhibitor, DIC, high blood pressure

262. Which of the following is a brand name for primidone?

    A. Prima
    B. Plendil
    C. Mysoline
    D. Probalan

263. Which of the following may be used as an antidote to benzodiazepine overdose?

I. Nalmefene
II. Physostigmine
III. Protamine
IV. Flumazenil

    A. I only
    B. II only
    C. I, II and III only
    D. IV only

264. Which of the following conditions is a contraindication for the use of NSAIDs?

    A. Hemoglobin levels over 14
    B. Evidence or history of GI bleeds
    C. A history of blood dyscrasias
    D. Joint pain

265. Which of the following would be considered a contraindication for the use of psyllium?

    A. Pregnancy.
    B. Hashimoto's thyroiditis
    C. Helminthic infection
    D. Intestinal obstruction

266. Which of the following forms is testosterone available in?

I. Injection
II. Topical gel
III. Subcutaneous implant
IV. Troche

    A. I only
    B. I, II and III only
    C. IV only
    D. Testosterone is available in all the listed forms.

267. Which of the following is potential side effect of niacin?

    A. Facial flushing
    B. Increased urination
    C. Decreased urination
    D. All of the above

268. **Which of the following are possible adverse effects of Folvite?**

I. Bronchospasm
II. Cardiac arrest
III. Tinnitus

    A. I only.
    B. II and III only
    C. I and III only
    D. All of the above are possible adverse effects.

269. **Which of the following statement(s) about A1c is/are TRUE?**

I. Measurement of A1c correlates approximately with the lifespan of a red blood cell, about 6-8 months.
II. Normal A1c should be at 4-6%.
III. A1c gives an approximation of glucose control in a patient corresponding to the previous 3-4 months.
IV. A1c will also be raised in chronic renal failure.

    A. I only
    B. II only
    C. II and III only
    D. II, III and IV only

270. **What is the mechanism of action of tolterodine (Detrol)?**

    A. Tolterodine is an opioid agonist.
    B. Tolterodine is a corticosteroid analog.
    C. Tolterodine is a GABA agonist.
    D. Tolterodine is an anti-cholinergic agent.

271. **Which of the following is an appropriate agent and dosing schedule for a newly diagnosed patient with depression?**

    A. Hydroxycobalamin, 200 mcg, PO, qd
    B. Venlafaxine, 37.5 mg, PO, bid
    C. Nortriptyline, 400 mg, PO, tid
    D. Ezetimide, 10 mg, PO, qd

Answers

1. **Answer: C** - Rhabdomyolysis is the rapid breakdown of skeletal muscle fiber and is associated with statin use. Mortality can rise to 20% in some patients. Asthenia, a known adverse effect of lovastatin, indicates muscular weakness and may be important as an early indication of rhabdomyolysis but is not, of itself, life-threatening. Pruritis is itching and is non-life-threatening. All of the above have been reported for lovastatin. The other most common adverse effects of lovastatin are headache, blurry vision, flatulence, dyspepsia, myalgia, cramping, abdominal pain and photosensitivity. A lupus-like syndrome has not been reported for lovastatin.

2. **Answer: D** - Bisphosphonates like Boniva (ibandronate sodium) are best absorbed on an empty stomach with a large amount of water to minimize gastrointestinal upset and esophageal irritation.

3. **Answer: C** - Clonazepam, when taken with Depacon (valproate), does increase the risk of absence seizures in patients with a history of absence seizure. Also, alcohol use increases the depressive effects of Depacon. Any patient on Depacon requires monitoring for neurologic status.

4. **Answer: A** - 2 mcg/min. 1 mg of epinephrine in 250 mL of solution = 0.004 mg/mL.(1 mg / 250 mL) At an infusion rate of 30 mL/hr, 0.12 mg will be infused every hour (0.004 mg/mL x 30 mL/hr). 0.12 mg/hr is equivalent to 0.002 mg/min (0.12 mg/hr x 1 hr / 60 min.). 0.002 mg/min is equivalent to 2 mcg/min (1mg = 1000 mcg).

5. **Answer: C** - Bisoprolol is a beta-adrenergic blocker. Busiperone is an anxiolytic. Budenoside is a corticosteroid. Phenoxybenzamine is an alpha-adrenergic blocker.

6. **Answer: A** - 50 mg of nitroglycerine in 250 mL of solution = 0.2 mg/mL (50 mg / 250 mL). At an infusion rate of 9 mL/hr, 1.8 mg will be infused every hour (0.2 mg/mL x 9 mL/hr). 1.8 mg/hr is equivalent to 0.03 mg/min (1.8 mg/hr x 1hr / 60min). 0.03 mg/min is equivalent to 30 mcg/min (1 mg = 1000mcg).

7. **Answer: A** - Clindamycin is the only one of the listed creams that is known to reduce the effectiveness of diaphragms and condoms, thereby decreasing the effectiveness of these birth control approaches.

8. **Answer: C** - Ambien is recommended only for short term use on the order of 7-10 days because of a risk of physical and psychological dependence. Sustiva (efavirenz) is a non-nucleoside reverse transcriptase inhibitor not known to cause dependence. Edrophonium is the generic name for Enlon, an anti-cholinesterase, also not known to cause dependence.

9. **Answer: B** - Metformin should not be given at more than 2000 mg each day. Glucose regulation often requires combinations of agents, and while blood sugars below 126 mg/dL are a reasonable goal, the maximum recommended dosages of hypoglycemic(s) should not be exceeded.

10. **Answer: D** - Vitamin B_{12} is the only water-soluble vitamin listed; Vitamins E, D and K are fat-soluble.

11. **Answer: A** - Decongestants are only approved by the FDA for allergic rhinitis and the common cold. Decongestants are NOT approved for sinusitis. Decongestants should not be used for children under 2 years of age.

12. **Answer: D** - Phenelzine should not be taken with food because it is an MOA (monoamine oxidase) inhibitor, and certain foods containing tyramine (cheese, yogurt, chocolate, soy, poultry and meats) should be avoided.

13. **Answer: B** - Iron is best absorbed in an acidic environment but can cause stomach upset on an empty stomach. Therefore the best advice is that iron should be given with food for maximum absorption and patient comfort.

14. **Answer: C** - Lithium is not associated with serious liver dysfunction or Stevens-Johnson syndrome. It is associated with a number of cardiac arrhythmias and circulatory collapse as well as seizures, syncope and coma.

15. **Answer: B** - Of the drugs listed, only Diovan HCT (Valsartan/Hydrochlorothiazide) is an anti-hypertensive and comes as a small pink oval pill. Amoxil (Amoxicillin) is an antibiotic, and the 500mg dose is a large pink tablet. Augmentin (200 mg) is a round pink pill and is a combination of amoxicillin and clavulanate K. Alprazolam/Xanax is an anxiolytic, and the 0.5 mg pill is oval, but not pink.

16. **Answer: B** - Vitamin B_2 can turn urine a bright yellow color. Vitamins A, D and E are fat-soluble and thereforeare not excreted in the urine.

17. **Answer: B** - Tegaserod (Zelnorm) is a partial 5HT4 agonist used to treat constipation in patients with IBS. Its use is contraindicated in gallbladder disease.

18. **Answer: B** - Trandolapril(Mavik) is a Category D drug and is contraindicated in pregnancy and lactation.

19. **Answer: D** - Lotrel os an antihypertensive combination of amlodipine and benzepril. Premphase is a conjugated estrogen/progestin combination. Vusion is a steroid free combination of miconazole and sodium bicarbonate used to treat diaper rash. Truvada is an anti-viral combination containing emtricitabine and tenofovir.

20. **Answer: C** - All of the listed drugs are associated with black box warnings. Tacrolimus has the potential for oto- and nephrotoxicity. Salmeterol has an increased risk of asthma-related death. Gadolimium-based contrast agents increase the risk of nephrogenic systemic fibrosis in patients with acute or chronic severe renal insufficiency. Tacrolimus has been associated with skin cancer and lymphoma.

21. **Answer: C** - Both statements A and B are correct.

22. **Answer: B** - Lansoprazole inhibits gastric acid secretion and is indicated for hyperacidity conditions. GERD (gastro esophageal reflux disease) and a duodenal ulcer would be indications for the use of lansoprazole. Crohn's disease and UC (ulcerative colitis) would not be indications.

23. **Answers: A and C** - 60mg PO q 4hrs means that two 30 mg capsules should be taken by mouth every 4 hours. PO means by mouth (per OS). Nimotop should be taken on an empty stomach.

24. **Answer: A** - Hydromorphone comes in 8 mg doses and is given in doses only up to 3-4mg every 4 hours. 80 mg every 4 hrs is an overdosing error. Hydromorphone is available as an injection, an oral solution, a rectal suppository and in a tablet form.

25. **Answer: D** - Melphalan is an alkylating agent and is known to induce thrombocytopenia. The treatment should be discontinued if the platelet count falls below 100,000/mm^3.

26. **Answer: D** - Tetracycline has known photosensitivity reactions. It also should NOT be taken with any milk or dairy products, antacids or laxatives. Prolonged therapy may induce a hemolytic anemia, neutropenia, thrombocytopenia and TTP.

27. **Answers: A and D** - A patient on a statin complaining of muscle cramping should have her liver function tested and CPK-MM tested for evidence of muscle damage. One of the serious adverse effects of a statin is rhabdomyolysis, and the patient's cramping may be symptomatic. CPK-MM levels are a good indicator of skeletal muscle damage occurring during rhabdomyolysis.

28. **Answer: B** - Mephyton is the brand name of phytonadione or Vitamin K and is used to treat the hypoprothrombinemia due to anti-coagulant therapy.

29. **Answer: D** - Minocycline, a tetracycline anti-infective used particularly in penicillin sensitive patients to treat gonorrhea, syphilis and acne, has all the listed as possible side effects.

30. **Answer: B** - Tobramycin is an anti-bacterial and interferes with protein synthesis. Ampicillin is another anti-bacterial and a beta-lactamase inhibitor. Clindamycin is a lincosamide anti-bacterial. Fluconasole is the only anti-fungal listed. Fluconazole is effective against *Candida* and *Cryptococcus* and can be used in children.

31. **Answer: C** - The most common and serious side effects of sulindac, a COX-1 enzyme inhibitor, are undetected GI bleeds and hyperkalemia (high serum potassium), which can lead to arrhythmias. Hyponatremia (low serum sodium) is not a known side effect of sulindac.

32. **Answer: C** - Sumatriptan is a selective 5HT$_1$ agonist and is a vascular headache suppressant. Etanercept is an anti-rheumatic agent, loxapine is an anti-psychotic and eptifibatide is an anti-platelet agent.

33. **Answer: C** - QVAR is a corticosteroid in an inhaled form and is only indicated for the treatment of asthma.

34. **Answer: B** - Simvastatin is an HMG-CoA reductase inhibitor. HMG-CoA reductase is the rate-limiting enzyme of the mevalonate (isoprenoid) pathway of cholesterol synthesis.

35. **Answer: C** - Saquinavir is a protease inhibitor (an antri-retroviral) and is used to treat HIV patients resistant to other antiretrovirals. Concurrent use of anti-arrhythmics can induce life-threatening reactions.

36. **Answer: D** - Eletriptan (Relpax) is a 5HT-1 receptor agonist and is used to treat migraines, but not basilar or hemiplegic migraines. A major contraindication is uncontrolled hypertension, and the most serious adverse reaction is cerebral or cardiovascular ischemia.

37. **Answer: A** - Phase I trials are usually small (N<20-30), but the aim is to determine the safe dose of a new drug.

38. **Answer: C** - Roferon-A is the trade name of recombinant interferon-alpha-2a. It is generally used in cases of hepatitis C and B. It is also an antineoplastic agent used to treat hairy cell leukemia, AIDS-related Kaposi's sarcoma and Ph[+] CML.

39. **Answer: B** - Hashimoto's thyroiditis is the most common form of hypothryroidism. Propylthiouracil is an anti-thyroid agent used to treat Grave's Disease (the most common form of hyperthyroidism) and would be contraindicated in Hashimoto's thyroiditis. Levothyroxine is synthetic T4. Cytomel is the brand name for Liothyronine (T3) Thyrolar contains both synthetic T4 and T3.

40. **Answer: B** - Azithromycin is effective against all the microbes listed and is most commonly used in community-acquired pneumonias, uncomplicated skin infectsion, pharyngitis and tonsillitis, COPD, PID and urethritis.

41. **Answer: D** - All of the statements are correct. Interferon-beta comes in an injectable form that should be refrigerated between uses. Rotating the areas for injection will minimize pain. NSAIDS are appropriate for the flu-like symptoms that often accompany IFN use. Patients must be monitored for mental health and for the arrhythmias, blood dyscrasias and intestinal obstructions that are the most serious reported side effects.

42. **Answer: C** - Rifabutin is marketed as Mycobutin, an anti-mycobacterila agent used to treat *Mycobacterium avium* in HIV[+] patients. Sandimmune, Gengraf and Neoral are brand names of cyclosporine.

43. **Answer: A** - Sulindac (Clinoril) is a COX-1 enzyme inhibitor and is contraindicated in asthma patients. Other contraindications include severe renal disease, 3rd trimester pregnancy and known hypersensitivity.

44. **Answer: D** - All the statements listed are accurate descriptions of UC and CD.

45. **Answer: B** - Statements II and III are the definitions of accuracy and precision. Neither accuracy nor precision relies on the dependent or the independent variables.

46. **Answer: D** - Quinolones should be avoided in patients with G6PD deficiency. The enzyme is found in red blood cells and protects against oxidative stress. African Americans have some of the highest rates of polymorphisms. There is no contraindication for the other listed agents.

47. **Answer: B** - Ondansetron (Zofran) is a 5HT3 antagonist. All of the listed drugs are used as anti-emetics in oncology. Aprepitant (Emend) is a neurokinin-1 antagonist. Metoclopramide (Reglan, Metazol, Octamide) is a dopamine-2 antagonist.

48. **Answer: D** - All the statements are true.

49. **Answer: C** - Hydroxyurea does not induce photosensitivity in sensitive individuals, though it may produce various skin reactions. The others listed all are known photosensitizing agents.

50. **Answer: C** - Rivastigmine is a cholinesterase inhibitor used to treat AD. A rare adverse effect is anxiety and tremor.

51. **Answer: C** - Ribavarin is a synthetic nucleoside analog and is an antiviral agent used primarily to treat refractory hepatitis C. Other main adverse effects include suicidal ideation, blood dyscrasias, pneumothorax, pancreatitis and other respiratory effects.

52. **Answer: B** - Etanercept is an immunomodulator used to treat moderate to severe RA and ankylosing spondylitis. In comes as an injection. Tolcapone is a catechol-O-methyltransferase (COMT) inhibitor and is used to treat Parkinson's disease. Topiramate blocks voltage dependent Na^+ channels and is used as an anti-seizure medication. Risdronate is a bisphosphonate used to treat osteoporosis.

53. **Answer: D** - Iron sucrose is used as an intravenous treatment of iron deficiency anemia. The other drug/delivery systems are correct; ferrous sulfate is the only oral preparation listed for the treatment of iron deficiency anemia.

54. **Answer: B** - NSAIDs inhibit prostaglandins via the cyclo-oxygenase pathway; therefore statement B is false. All other statements are true.

55. **Answer: A** - The "B" in the gold-standard antineoplastic combination ABVD is for bleomycin. The other drugs in the combination are Adriamycin, vinblastine and dacarbazine. Baclofen is a SM relaxant. Bivalirudin is an anticoagulant. Buspirone is an anxiolytic.

56. **Answer: C** - Patients on Imuran (azathiaprine) should be monitored for pancreatic enzyme levels (amylase and lipase), LFTs and CBCs. The most common adverse reactions include blood dyscrasias, serum sickness and hepatotoxicity.

57. **Answer: A** - Pyrazinamide, a niacinamide derivative, is used to treat tuberculosis. Celcoxib is marketed as Celebrex and is a non-steroidal COX-s inhibitor used to treat OA and RA. Propoxyphene, marketed as Darvon, is a non-opioid analgesic.

58. **Answer: D** - In choices I, II and III, the drugs are correctly paired with the mechanism of action. Donepazil is an acetylcholinesterase inhibitor used to treat Alzheimer's disease.

59. **Answer: D** - None of the agents listed are anti-arrhythmic agents. Ondansetron (Zofran) is a 5HT3 antagonist. Filgrastim (Neupogen) is a leukocyte colony stimulating factor. Zolpidem (Ambien) is a sedative-hypnotic agent.

60. **Answer: A** - Cholecalciferol is another term for Vitamin D3. It is contraindicated in cases of hypercalcemia. Thromboembolic events are not associated with Vitamin D use.

61. **Answer: C** - A bilateral orchiectomy and/or the use of an LH-RH antagonist are considered to be effective therapy for prostate cancer. Testosterone antagonists alone are not considered an effective therapy.

62. **Answer: D** - Mycophenolate mofetil is a mycophenolic acid derivative and inhibits the binding of IL-1, thereby suppressing the immune response.

63. **Answer: A** - Botulinum toxin A (Botox) is the only neuromuscular blocker and is non-depolarizing. Oxcabazepine (Oxetal) is a mood stabilizer and anti-convulsant and blocks voltage-sensitive sodium channels. Chlordiazepoxide (Librium) is a benzodiazepine anxiolytic that binds to GABA receptors, potentiating its effects. Finasteride (Proscar, Propecia, Fincar, Finpecia, Finax, Finast, Finara, Finalo, Prosteride, Gefina, Appecia) is an androgen inhibitor used in BPH and male-pattern baldness.

64. **Answer: D** - Bipolar disorder is most often treated with mood stabiliziers such as lithium or lamotrigine. Aripiprazole is an antipsychotic/neuroleptic with partial agonist activity at D2 and 5HT-1A receptors. Azothiaprine is an anti-rheumatic disease-modifying agent. Zoledronic acid is a calcium regulator, but it is not used in the treatment of bipolar disorder.

65. **Answer: D** - Amitriptyline is a tricyclic antidepressant and not an antipsychotic. All the other drugs listed are considered atypical antipsychotics.

66. **Answer: D** - In the anemia of chronic kidney disease, the red blood cells are NOT macrocytic, but are normocytic-of normal size. This would also mean a normal MCV. Statements II, III and IV are true for anemia of chronic kidney disease.

67. **Answer: C** - Avapro is the brand name for irbesartan, an angiotensin II receptor antagonist (antihypertensive). Nimotop is the brand name for mimodipine, a calcium channel blocker (antihypertensive). Plendil (felodipine) is also a calcium channel blocker used to treat hypertension. Plaquenil (hydroxychloroquine) is an antimalarial drug also used to treat systemic lupus erythematosis and rheumatoid arthritis.

68. **Answer: A** - Heparin is incompatible with insulin in an IV infusion. The other agents listed may be given along with insulin.

69. **Answer: D** - Docusate is a laxative. Intestinal obstruction is considered a contraindication for the use of any laxative. Hip dysplasia, IDDM (Insulin Dependent Diabetes Mellitus) and pregnancy are not contraindications for laxative use.

70. **Answer: D** - Miperidine is an analgesic opioid agonist. All the drugs listed except miperidine are used to treat tuberculosis.

71. **Answer: A** - Carbidopa is a dopa-decarboxylase inhibitor and thus prevents levodopa degradation by that enzyme in the periphery (levodopa is a dopamine analog). The other statements are not true.

72. **Answer: B** - Methimazole is an anti-thyroid agent used in hyperthyroidism and comes only in tablet form.

73. **Answer: D** - Ramipil is the generic name for Altace, an ACE inhibitor. Zonizamide (a sulfonamide) is the generic name of Zonegran. Lovastatin, an HMG-CoA reductase inhibitor, is the generic name of Altocor and Mevacor. Lisinopril, another ACE inhibitor, is the generic name of Prinivil or Zestril.

74. **Answer: D** - All the conditions listed are potential side effects of lovastatin use. Lovastatin is an HMG-CoA reductase inhibitor used to tread hypercholesterolemia and other hyperlipidemias.

75. **Answer: D** - Methotrexate is a folic acid antagonist used as an immunosuppressant and an antineoplastic agent. All of the listed adverse effects are possible with methotrexate use.

76. **Answer: D** - Methotrexate is a Pregnancy category X medication; the use of contraception by women of reproductive age is required. Rivastigmine is a cholinesterase inhibitor and is a Pregnancy Category B drug. Dronobinol is a cannabinoid analog used as an antiemetic and is also a Pregnancy Category B drug. Infliximab in a monoclonal antibody used to treat rheumatoid arthritis and is a Pregnancy Category C agent.

77. **Answer: C** - Boniva (ibandronate), Inderide (a combination of HCTZ and propranolol) and OxyContin (a slow-release form of oxycodone) should never be crushed, as they are all timed-released. Propylthiouracil, an anti-thyroid agent, may be crushed.

78. **Answer: A** - A1c does correlate with the lifespan of a red blood cell (rbc), but the lifespan of an rbc is on the order of 3-4 months (90-120 days) and NOT 6-8 months. The other statements are true.

79. **Answer: D** - Bumetanide is a loop diuretic. The other agents listed are all anti-arrhythmics.

80. **Answer: D** - Benzapril and ramipril are both ACE (angiotensisn converting enzyme) inhibitors. Losartan in an angiotensin II receptor antagonist.

81. **Answer: D** - Allopurinol is the only anti-gout agent listed, and the dosage listed is possible. Acarbose is a hypoglycemic, and the dose listed is possible. Alitretinoin is a topical antineoplastic and may be used up to 4 times a day. Hydroxycobalamin is Vitamin B_{12}, and the dosage listed is possible.

82. **Answer: A** - The "B" in the gold-standard antineoplastic combination BEAM, used in non-Hodgkin's Lymphoma (NHL), is BCNU or carmustine, an alkylating agent. The M is for melpahlan, a mustard derivative,

83. **Answer: C** - The trade name of rifaxamin is Xifaxan. It is an anti-infective used most often to treat traveller's diarrhea. The others are correctly matched.

84. **Answer: A** - Itracozanole is an anti-fungal agent that prevents ergosterol synthesis in fungal cell membranes. It is used in aspergillosis, blastomycosis and histoplasmosis.

85. **Answer: D** - All of the listed adverse effects are possible with the use of pindolol.

86. **Answer: D** - Vitamin K, a phylloquinone, is also known as phytonadione and is used to treat hypoprothrombinemia caused by the use of anti-coagulants.

87. **Answer: D** - Nifedipine is a calcium channel blocker. Moricizine is a sodium channel blocker.
Modafinil is a CNS stimulant. Aripiprazole is an antipsychotic.

88. **Answer: B** - Repaglinide is an alpha-glucosidase inhibitor used to treat NIDDM. Adverse effects include hyper- and hypo-glycemia.

89. **Answer: D** - Sulfisoxazole is a sulfonamide anti-infective. Two possible adverse effects are psudomembranous colitis (with diarrhea) and pneumonitis and pulmonary infiltrates (SOB, dyspnea). Hypertension is not a likely adverse reaction.

90. **Answer: B** - Alendronate is a bisphosphonate. Methotrexate is a folic acid inhibitor. Ribavarin is an antiviral nucleoside analog. Orlistat is a GI lipase inhibitor.

91. **Answer: A** - Orlistat is a GI lipase inhibitor marketed as Xenical. The other names are made up.

92. **Answer: D** - Sildenafil is a type 5 phosphodiesterase inhibitor used to treat erectile dysfunction. Verapamil is a calcium channel blocker. Furosemide is a loop diuretic. Budenoside is a corticosteroid.

93. **Answer: C** - All the drugs listed are removed during hemodialysis. Levels of medications should be monitored in patients who are undergoing dialysis.

94. **Answer: C** - All the drugs listed are removed during peritoneal dialysis. Levels of medications should be monitored in patients who are undergoing dialysis.

95. **Answer: B** - Renal, hepatic or heart disease would be considered precautionary for the use of inamrinone, an inotropic vasodilator generally suited for the short-term management of heart failure.

96. **Answer: A** - Thiazide diuretics (or diuretics in general) are often considered the first line of therapy in mild-moderate hypertension.

97. **Answer: D** - All the drugs listed are bronchodilators.

98. **Answer: C** - All the drugs listed except mirtazapine, an antidepressant, are bronchodilators and may be used to treat asthma.

99. **Answer: B** - Cyclosporine is available as an IV, capsule and oral solution.

100. **Answer: B** - Ofloxacin is a fluoroquinolone and inhibits bacterial DNA synthesis by inhibiting the DNA gyrase. It is commonly used in infections of the GU tract, eyes and ears.

101. **Answer: B** - Sumatriptan is a selective 5HP-1 agonist and is used to treat acute migraines.

102. **Answer: A** - Sumatriptan is a selective 5HP-1 agonist . Vasospasm and MI are both potential adverse events associated with sumatriptan.

103. **Answer: A** - Danazol is a synthetic androgen used to treat mild to moderate endometriosis and fibrocystic disease. It is contraindicated in abnormal bleeding, porphyria, severe hepatic, renal or cardiac disease and pregnancy/lactation.

104. **Answer: C** - Allopurinol and colchicine are used both as prophylactics and in treatment of acute gout. NSAIDs and corticosteroids are not prophylactic for gout, but are used for pain treatment of an acute crisis.

105. **Answer: A** - Orlistat is a GI lipase inhibitor used to treat obesity along with a calorie-restricted diet. Lepirudin is an anti-coagulant. The dose given is appropriate. Lovastatin is an antihyperlipidemic. The dosing schedule given is appropriate. Ranitidine is a histamine-2 receptor antagonist, and the dosing schedule listed would be appropriate for acute duodenal ulcer.

106. **Answer: B** - Oral antibiotics interfere with the efficacy of oral contraceptives, and a backup method of contraception is strongly recommended. It would be incorrect and ethically wrong to recommend stopping contraceptive use or doubling up on the oral contraceptive.

107. **Answer: D** - With bp> 240/130 and with end organ involvement evident, current guidelines recommend nitroprusside IV (0.1 mcg/kg/min). The other agents listed are used in less critical situations.

108. **Answer: B** - The "N" in the TNM staging system represents nodal involvement. The "T" represents the severity of the primary or main tumor. "M" represents the presence or absence of distant metastases.

109. **Answer: C** - Gleevec is the brand name of imatinib. The others are correctly matched. Gleevec is a tyrosine-kinase inhibitor, specifically the Bcr-Abl protein found in most patients with CML.

110. **Answer: B** - Univasc/moexipril is an ACE inhibitor. Aripiprazole is an atypical antipsychotic. Piroxicam is an NSAID. Edrophonium is a cholinesterase inhibitor.

111. **Answer: C** - Pyridostigmine, used to treat myesthenia gravis, is an anti-cholinesterase and is available in all the forms listed.

112. **Answer: D** - Entacapone is a COMT-inhibitor used as an adjunct in Parkinson's disease. Albuterol is a bronchodilator. Zoledronic acid is a bisphosphonate, and liotrix is a synthetic T3 analog.

113. **Answer: A** - Tolbutamide is a hypoglycemic agent used to treat non-insulin-dependent diabetes mellitus (Type 2). A serious adverse event is the development of the syndrome of inappropriate antidiuretic hormone secretion (SIADH).

114. **Answer: D** - A K^+ sparing diuretic is often the first line to treat mild to moderate hypertension by inhibiting reabsorption of electrolytes in proximal and distal tubules and in the loop of Henle. Glucose is not normally affected. Blood pressure and electrolytes should be monitored to determine the effectiveness and safety of any diuretics.

115. **Answer: B** - All the agents listed are vasodilators and act by stimulating the intracellular production of cGMP.

116. **Answer: D** - Immunosuppressants are contraindicated in severe infection and in pregnant patients with rheumatoid arthritis (RA). Caution is advised in uncompensated heart failure.

117. **Answer: D** - Topical corticosteroids are effective in the treatment of psoriasis. Basilixamab is an immunosuppressant. Topotecan and Paclitaxl are antineoplastics.

118. **Answer: B** - When studying 2 groups, the paired t-tests would be appropriate. ANOVA (analysis of variance between groups) would be the preferred test for numerical data with 3 or more groups. Mann-Whitney is a non-parametric test, and chi-square tests are used on nominal (coded) data.

119. **Answer: B** - Alendronate is a bisphosphonate. Carmustine is an alkylating agent. Etoposide is a pdodphyllotoxin. Gemcitabine is an anti-metabolite.

120. **Answer: C** - Lexxel is an antihypertensive combination containing enalapril and felodipine. Emtricitambine/disoproxil (Truvada) is an antiviral. HCTZ/Losartan is Hyzaar, an anti-hypertensive. Amylase, lipase and protease is sold as Ultrase, digestive enzymes.

121. **Answer: C** - Galantamaine (reminyl) is used to treat mild to moderater Alzheimer's disease. It is a cholinesterase inhibitor.

122. **Answer: C** - All are possible signs and symptoms of respiratory alkalosis.

123. **Answer: A** - Agranulocytemia is characterized by chills, fever, malaise and fatigue, not by hallucinations.

124. **Answer: D** - Venlafaxine (Effexor) is available as an extended release capsule and tablet and is not given as an IM.

125. **Answer: B** - PSA is normally < 4 ng/mL. For a value > 50ng/mL, prostatitis and prostate cancer must be ruled out.

126. **Answer: C** - Alfentanil is an opioid analgesic. Enalapril and lisinopril are renin-angiotensin antagonists and used to treat hypertension.

127. **Answer: C** - Thiopental is used for the slow induction of anesthesia as well as for its maintenance. Ropivicaine is used in lumbar blocks. Pancuronium is used to relax skeletal muscles for intubation. Fentenyl is used for short-term analgesia.

128. **Answer: B** - Endocet is a combination of acetaminophen and oxycodone and is used for pain relief. Atamet is a carbidopa/levodopa combination used in PA. Epzicom is an antiviral containing abacavir and lamivudine. Zestoretic is an antihypertensive comtaining HCTZ and lisinopril.

129. **Answer: C** - Irbesartan is an angiotensin II receptor antagonist used to treat hypertension.

130. **Answer: B** - Nateglinide stimulates the secretion of insulin from pancreatic beta cells. Paroxetine is an antidepressant. Tocainide is an anti-arrhythmic. Magnesium oxide is an antacid.

131. **Answer: D** - While normal lab values vary for clinic to clinic, all the above values would be considered within normal limits.

132. **Answer: C** - The patient's mass must be taken into account particularly for dopamine infusion. For the other agents, the rate is dependent on the dosage desired.

133. **Answer: A** - Valtrex, 1000 mg is a large, dark blue tablet. Amoxicillin, 875 mg is a large pink tablet. Zocor, 80 mg is a dusty rose tablet, and venlafaxine is a pink pentagon.

134. **Answer: A** - Olanzipine (Zyprexa) is an antipsychotic, believed to antagonize dopamine and serotonin receptors centrally and muscarinic receptors in the periphery. It is used to treat schizophrenia, bipolar disorder and acute manic episodes. Other major adverse effects include lukopenia, hyperglycemia and coma.

135. **Answer: C** - Angioedema (aka angioneurotic edema) is a vascular dilatory reaction. It is not a symptom of anaphylaxis.

136. **Answer: B** - Red yeast rice naturally contains mevinic acid or lovastatin.

137. **Answer: D** - Vecuronium is a neuromuscular blocker (non-depolarizing), a competitive inhibitor of acetylcholine. Milrinone is an inotropic agent. Amlodipine is a Ca^{2+} channel blocker, and finasteride is a 5 α-reductase inhibitor.

138. **Answer: A** - Olanzapine is marketed as Zyprexa or Zydis. Lanza and Quiettime are made up names. Prozac is the brand name of fluoxetine

139. **Answer: B** - Leucovorin allows DNA replication to continue in healthy cells by providing an alternative folic acid source independent of dihydrofolate reductase. Since methotrexate is a dihydrofolate reductase inhibitor, leukovorin can provide a "rescue." Doxorubicin is an intercalating agent, and cytarabine is an inhibitor or DNA polymerase. There is no overlap in the mechanisms, and leucovorin would not rescue any of those two treatments.

140. **Answer: A** - A child older than 4 years old can get a maintenance dose and should get 0.4mg (= 400 mcg) per day either PO, IM or sc. The other doses given are too high.

141. **Answer: C** - Tamoxifen is available only as a tablet form and an oral solution. It is a non-steroidal anti-estrogen used as an adjunct to breast cancer treatment as well,as a preventive treatment for women at high risk for breast cancer and for the treatment of ductal CIS.

142. **Answer: A** - Plaquenil is the brand name of hydroxyquinolone, used to treat and prevent malaria and to treat rheumatoid arthritis and SLE. Quinapril (Accupril) is an ACE inhibitor. Quinate is a Canadian brand name for quinidine, used as an anti-malarial and an anti-arrhythmic. Quixin is a brand name for levofloxacin, a fluroquinone anti-infective.

143. **Answer: B** - Prazosin (Minipress) is an α-adrenergic blocker (peripherally acting) and is used to treat hypertension (and off-label, benign prostatic hypertrophy (BPH)).

144. **Answer: A** - Tenecteplase is a thrombolytic used to reduce the mortality associated with MIs. It has serious adverse effects including hemorrhage, cardiogenic shock, re-infarction, heart failure and other CV effects.

145. **Answer: A** - Saw palmetto (*Serenoa repens*) is used to treat benign prostatic hypertrophy and has been shown to have inhibitory activity against 5-α-reductase, thereby inhibiting testosterone production.

146. **Answer: A** - Hydrocodone (eg Lortab) and and Sertraline (Zoloft) are two of the most common drugs prescribed. Sargramostim (Leukine) is a granulocyte-macrophage stimulating factore used to stimulate blood cell production after chemotherapy or transplantation.

147. **Answer: C** - Gleevec (imatinib) is a tyrosine kinase inhibitor used specifically for CML (after the failure of IFN therapy) and in CD117+ GI stromal tumors.

148. **Answer: A** - Ketoprofen (Actron) is an NSAID that (presumably) inhibits prostaglandin and leukotriene synthesis and is used to treat RA, OA and primary dysmennorrhea and as an anti-pyretic.

149. **Answer: B** - Cyanocobalamin is the chemical name for Vitamin B_{12}. Phytonadione is the term for Vitamin K. Cholecalciferol is Vitamin D_3 and Pyridoxine is VitaminB_6.

150. **Answer: B** - All the other agents listed except albuterol are diuretics. Albuterol is a bronchodilator. Acetazolamide is a carbonic anhydrase inhibitor. Mannitol is an osmotic diuretic, and metolazone is a thiazide diuretic.

151. **Answer: D** - Tramadol (Ultram) is an opioid agonist and used as an analgesic in moderate to severe pain. As with all opioids, a serious adverse effect is respiratory depression.

152. **Answer: A** - All the complications listed are possible with tretinoin use. Other adverse effects include multiple organ failure, hepatosplenomegaly, MIs and renal failure. Tretinoin is an antineoplastic dermatologic agent used to treat acute promyelocytic leukemias, acne vulgaris and for cosmetic purposes.

153. **Answer: A** - Grapefruit juice interferes with Phase I Liver detoxification processes, specifically with the CYP450 isoform, CYP3A4.

154. **Answer: B** - Lanoxin is the brand name for digoxin and is generally used to treat heart failure, tachyarrhythmias, fibrillations and flutters.

155. **Answer: A** - Duloxetine is an SSRI and an antidepressant. Use of alcohol should be discouraged as it does increase the risk of liver damage. There is no reported increased risk of bleeding when used with warfarin.

156. **Answer: B** - Indinavir is an anti-retroviral protease inhibitor and is used for HIV infection. All the other anti-virals listed are not useful in an infection with an RNA virus.

157. **Answer: D** - Vytorin is an antihyperlipidemic and consists of ezetimide and simvastatin. Vusion is the combination of miconazole with $NaHCO_3$ and is used to treat diaper dermatitis. Carbidopa and levodopa combined are marketed as Cinemet, which is used to treat PD. HCTZ combined with propranolol is marketed as Inderide for the treatment of hypertension.

158. **Answer: A** - Zyrtec-D is a combination of cetirizine and pseudoephedrine. The main potentially serious side effects are bronchospasm and angioedema.

159. **Answer: B** - Dalteparin/Fragmin is a low molecular weight heparin and is used to block clot formations.

160. **Answer: D** - All of the listed adverse effects are possible with phenazopyridine, Bright orange urine is the most common.

161. **Answer: B** - Nizatidine (Axid) is an H-2 receptor antagonist and is used to decrease gastric acid secretion.

162. **Answer: A** - Lotrel (amlodipine/benzapril- antihypertensive) comes as a capsule (2.5/10 mg, 5/10 mg, 5/20 mg, 10/20 mg). Norvasc is a white tablet (2.5 mg, 5 mg, 10 mg). Xanax is a tablet (.025 mg, 0.5 mg, 1 mg, 2 mg). Fosamax is a white tablet (5 mg, 10 mg, 35 mg, 70 mg).

163. **Answer: B** - Alprazolam is metabolized via the CYP3A4. Warfarin is metabolized via the CYP2C9 pathway. Theophylline is metabolized via the CYP1A2; fluoxetine, via the CYP2D6 pathway. These pathways are particularly important to be aware of because of drug interactions, leading to increased or decrease serum concentrations.

164. **Answer: B** - Catapres patches are applied weekly and the patient should overlap the two delivery systems in order to maintain effective drug levels. A patient should not be advised to stop taking the medication immediately. The Catapres patch has been shown to be effective and to increase patient compliance.

165. **Answer: A** - OTC products with caffeine may exacerbate migraines. Anti-depressants may be used as prevention (prophylaxis) for migraines and OTC migraine analgesics may treat migraines symptomatically, but they are not indicated for prevention. Anti-hypertensives may have some effect in migraines where hypertension places a role but are not generally used as a prophylactic treatment for migraine.

166. **Answer: C** - Droperidol is an anti-emetic and used for post-operative nausea and vomiting. Dolora is an opioid analgesic used for moderate to severe pain. Fentora and Actiq are used for breakthrough pain in cancer patients tolerant to opioids.

167. **Answer: B** - Phenobarbital is available in all the listed forms except timed-release tablets.

168. **Answer: D** - Clopidogrel is the only anti-platelet agent listed. It inhibits platelet aggregation by preventing binding to the glycoprotein receptor, GPIIb/IIIa. Inamrinone is an inotropic agent. Benzotropine is an ant-cholinergic. Busulfan is an alkylating agent.

169. **Answer: A** - Cholestyramine is water-soluble bile acid sequestrant and a lipid-lowering medication. It may be taken with food or water. It should not be mixed with any carbonated beverage as this decreases absorption.

170. **Answer: C** - 5 HT-3 receptor antagonists are used as anti-nausea and anti-emetic agents. Fluroquinolones are anti-infectives. MAO inhibitors increase dopaminergic activity. HMG-CoA reductase inhibitors are anti-hyperlipidemic agents.

171. **Answer: A** - Glipizide (Glucotrol) is a hypoglycemic agent in the sufonylurea class and is indicated for non-insulin dependent diabetes (NIDDM). Sirolimus (Rapamune) is a lactone used most often as an immunosuppressant in transplant patients. Tiotropium is an anit-muscarinic/anti-cholinergic bronchodilator. Olmesartan (Benicar) is an angiotensin II inhibitor used in treating hypertension.

172. **Answer: A** - Liothyronine is a synthetic thyroid hormone replacement and is an analog to T3. Since Graves' disease is hyperthyroid, the patient is producing too much T3/T4, and more should not be given.

173. **Answer: D** - The macrolides, barbiturates and rotinavir all have known interactions with oral contraceptives, interfering with Phase I and Phase II reactions. Macrolides, anti-retrovirals and barbiturates are all associated with decreased oral contraceptive efficacy.

174. **Answer: A** - Olmesartan (Benicar) is an angiotensin II receptor antagonist and is an anti-hypertenisve. Glipizide (Glucotrol) is a hypoglycemic agent in the sufonylurea class and is indicated for non-insulin dependent diabetes (NIDDM). Repaglinide is also a hypoglycemic and is an alpha-glucosidase inhibitor marketed as Prandin. Sirolimus (Rapamune) is an immunosuppressant.

175. **Answer: D** - Cholestyramine is a bile acid sequestrant and lowers serum lipids. It is used to treat biliary obstructions.

176. **Answer: B** - Bisphosphonates are best absorbed on an empty stomach with a large amount of water to minimize gastrointestinal upset and esophageal irritation.

177. **Answer: D** - Both carbemazepine and lamotrigine are anti-convulsants. Fondaparinux is an anto-coagulant.

178. **Answer: A** - Exubera is the brand name for the powdered, inhalable form of insulin. Humulin is an isophane, long-acting injectable form. Lantus is also a long acting insulin form given by injection. NovoLog is a short-acting insulin given by injections.

179. **Answer: C** - Ticlodipine is a platelet aggregation inhibitor. Pyrazinamide is an anti-tubercular medication. Etanercept is a biological response modifier used to treat RA. Ziprasidone is an antipsychotic.

180. **Answer: C** - Moricizine is a sodium channel blocker used to treat ventricular arrhythmias. Arrhythmias and thrombophlebitis are potential side effects. Psuedomembranous colitis is associated with the use of certain anti-infectives and not with sodium channel blockers. Moricizine is also associated with adverse cerebrovascular events.

181. **Answer: A** - Selegiline (Eldepryl) is an MAOI used to treat major depressive disorder and PD. Sotalol is a beta-adrenergic nonselective bloker. Trazodone is an anti-depressant. Sorafenib is a multi-kinase inhibitor/antineoplastic.

182. **Answer: C** - Moricizine is an anti-arrhythmic agent. ECGs, fluid balance and blood pressure levels should all be carefully monitored. Bowel movements, while important, would not be considered vital in this patient.

183. **Answer: B** - Amlodipine is a calcium channel blocker used to treat hypertension. Bethanechol is a cholinergic used to treat urinary spasm or retention. Benzapril is an ACE inhibitor and another anti-hypertensive agent. Alfentanil is an opioid analgesic.

184. **Answer: D** - Monteleukast is marketed as Singulair and is a leukotriene receptor antagonist, indicated in long-term asthma management.

185. **Answer: A** - Humulin is an isophane insulin. Isophane refers to a crystalline suspension of insulin, protamine and zinc used for injection. The isophane insulins are long-acting insulins. Humulog (lispro) is a short-acting insulin. Novolog is a recombinant, short-acting insulin. Ultralente is a very short-acting insulin.

186. **Answer: C** - Maxzide is a combination of hydrochlorothiazide (HCTZ) and triamterene used to treat hypertension. Amiloride plus HCTZ is known as Moduretic and is a diuretic. Quibron is a combination of guaifenisin and theophylline used to induce bronchodilation.

187. **Answer: A** - Naratriptan is indicated for migraines and NOT basilar headaches.

188. **Answer: B** - Psoriasis is treated using topical vitamin D analogs. Calcipotriene (Dovonex), for example, is a cream, ointment or solution containing a vitamin D analog used to treat mild to moderate psoriasis.

189. **Answer: A** - 1 gram is equal to 15.43 grains (or ~15 ½ grains) A grain is a measurement of mass, while minim and a fluid ounce are measurements of volume.

190. **Answer: B** - Pseudophedrine/Drixoral is a sympathomimetic, and as such, it should be used with caution in a patient with hyperthyroidism or glaucoma. Psuedophedrine is generally prescribed for nasal or sinus congestion.

191. **Answer: A** - Tzmoxifen comes as an oral soulution (10mg/5mL) and as tablets (10 mg, 20 mg). 200 mg represents a 10-fold overdose. The prescriber must be called and informed of the mistake. Tamoxifen can cause DVT and pulmonary emboli as well as blood dyscrasias. It is unethical to dispense as written without checking or to simply document your concerns.

192. **Answer: D** - All of the listed adverse events except for hyperkalemia and hyponatremia are associated with Xanax (alprazolam) use and must be discussed with the woman. Given that she wants to get pregnant and that abrupt withdrawal is not recommended, an alternative antidepressant should also be discussed.

193. **Answer: A** - The FDA does not recommend the use of decongestants in children under 6. Pseudophedrine is used OTC in Dimetapp, Sudafed and Triaminic. Psyllium is a bulk laxative. Sirolimus is a macrocyclic lactone immunosuppressant, and sulfisoxazole is a short-acting sulfonamide anti-infective.

194. **Answer: C** - Celecoxib/Celebrex, a COX-2 inhibitor, carries the increased risk of thrombotic, GI and cardiac events. Ibuprofen, an NSAID also carries the increased risk of thrombotic, GI and cardiac events. ACE inhibitors, as a class, can cause injury and death to a developing fetus. Acarbose is a hypoglycemic and carries no black box warning.

195. **Answer: A** - A is a correct statement. Neseritide (Natracor) is a B-type natriuretic peptide vasodilator and is contraindicated in obstructive cardiomyopathy and in hypotensive patients with systolic pressures less than 90 mm Hg. Bosentan (Tracleer) is an endothelin-receptor agonist (not an ACE inhibitor) and should be used cautiously in patients with mitral stenosis or pulmonary hypertension and with elderly patients. LFT are required with bosentan use.

196. **Answer: B** - Minoxidil is a vasodilator and is used to treat hypertension. All the other drugs listed are used to treat rheumatoid arthritis (RA).

197. **Answer: D** - All the drugs listed are inhibitors of the CYP2D6 pathway and can interact with other medications to produce serious adverse effects by increasing the serum concentrations of drugs metabolized by the CYP2D6 pathway.

198. **Answer: B** - Prostimin (neostigmine) is an anticholinesterase used to treat MG. It is available both as an injection and in tablet form. As an anticholinesterase, a cholinergic crisis is a potential adverse effect, and atropine should be readily available. Prostigmin is generally given on an inpatient basis; self-administration is not usually required.

199. **Answer: D** - Glucotrol comes as a 5mg or 10 mg extended-release tablet and should be swallowed (not crushed or dissolved) and be taken 30 minutes before breakfast.

200. **Answer: A** - 8 drahms (alternative spelling: dram) is equal to 1 fluid ounce.

201. **Answer: B** - 1 drahm is equal to 1.3 U.S. teaspoons.

202. **Answer: A** - Vitamins C, the B-complex vitamins and the beta-carotenes are water-soluble. vitamin A (and vitamins D, E and K) are fat-soluble vitamins.

203. **Answer: C** - According to the National Coordinating Council for Medication Error Reporting and Prevention (NCC MERP), it is crucial that "health care professionals administer only medications that are properly labeled and that during the administration process, labels be read three times: when reaching for or preparing the medication, immediately prior to administering the medication, and when discarding the container or replacing it into its storage location."

204. **Answer: C** - Cerebyx is the brand name for fosphenytoin, an anticonvulsant. Celebrex is the brand name for celecoxib, a COX-2 inhibitor and an NSAID. Celexa is the brand name for citalopram, an SSRI.

205. **Answer: A** - Clonidine (Catapres) is a centrally acting sympatholytic. Klonopin is the brand name for clonazepam, a benzodiazepine. The trade name Klonopin can easily be confused with the generic name clonidine. Norpramin is the brand name for desipramine, a TCA.

206. **Answer: C** - Zyprexa is the brand name of olanzapine, a thienebenzodiazepine anti-psychotic medication. Zyvox is the brand name of linezolid, an anti-infective. Zyrtec is the brand name of cetirizine, an H_1 receptor antagonist.

207. **Answer: D** - Pseudomembranous colitis is a classic adverse effect of clindamycin use, and potentially the most serious. Neutropenia and hepatic dysfunction are also possible adverse effects.

208. **Answer: A** - "qd" is no longer recommended. Instead, one should write out, "every day."

209. **Answer: B** - The Joint Commission for medication safety recommends the use of a "leading zero" to ensure the decimal point is recognized.

210. **Answer: B** - 500 mcg is the correct form; the greek letter "μ" is no longer used in hand-writing medication because of potential reading erors. Choice "C" is incorrect because the Joint Commission for medication safety recommends the use of a "leading zero" to ensure the decimal point is recognized.

211. **Answer: A** - Metronidazole (Flagyl) is an anti-protozoal agent. Metfomin (Glucophage) is a hypoglycemic. Metopolol (Toprol-XL or Lopressor) is a beta-blocker, and metolazone is a thiazide diuretic.

212. **Answer: B** - Tetracycline should NOT be taken with any milk or dairy products, antacids or laxatives, and no drug should be taken within 1hr of alcohol ingestion. Tetracycline has known photosensitivity reactions and is best taken with large amounts of water on an empty stomach.

213. **Answer: D** - A patient on a statin complaining of muscle cramping should have his liver function tested and CPK-MM tested for evidence of muscle damage. One of the serious adverse effects of a statin is rhabdomyolysis, and the patient's cramping may be symptomatic. CPK-MM levels are a good indicator of skeletal muscle damage occurring during rhabdomyolysis.

214. **Answer: C** - The abbreviation "qid" means four times a day. It is an abbreviation for "quater in die."

215. **Answer: C** - 15 U.S. minims is approximately equal to 1 millileter (mL), which is equal to 1 cc (cubic centimeter).

216. **Answer: A** - Probenecid (Benemid) and Allopurinol (Lopurin, Zyloprim) are anti-hyperuricemic (anti-gout) agents. Dobutamine (Dobutrex) is a positive inotrope.

217. **Answer: D** - Entecavir (Baraclude) is a guanosine nucleoside analog and an antiviral used to threat chronic hepatitis B infections. All the listed adverse effects are possible with entecavir use.

218. **Answer: A** - Azithromycin in a high dose is effective against *Moraxella catarrhalis Moraxella catarrhalis* is a gram negative organism and produces beta-lactamase. Penicillins such as ampicillin and amoxicillin are ineffective against gram negative bacteria. Fluconasole is an azole antifungal.

219. **Answer: A** - Clindamycin is a lincosamide anti-infective and has activity mainly against aerobic Gram (-) rods such as *Bacteroides* and Gram (+) cocci such as *Staphylococcus.* It is not effective against *Psuedomonas*. One of the serious side effects of clindamycin (Cleocin, Dalacin C) use is *Clostridiadifficile* overgrowth and potential pseudomembranous colitis.

220. **Answer: D** - QVAR (beclomethasone) is an inhaled form of corticosteroid and is indicated for the treatment of asthma and rhinitis.

221. **Answer: A** - A spirometer (blow tube) is used to measure the lung's forced vital capacity. A sphygmomanometer measures blood pressure, and a goniometer measures angles in range of motion tests. A nebulizer is used for inhalation therapy, not measurement.

222. **Answer: D** - All of the listed drugs are used as anti-emetics in oncology. Aprepitant (Emend) is a neurokinin-1 antagonist. Ondansetron (Zofran) and Palonosetron (Aloxi) are $5HT_3$ receptor antagonists. Metoclopramide (Reglan, Metazol, Octamide) is a dopamine-2 antagonist.

223. **Answer: B** - A sphygmomanometer measures blood pressure. A caliper is a tool used to measure distance or length. A spirometer (blow tube) is used to measure forced vital capacity and other respiratory parameters. A Grave's speculum is a type of vaginal speculum.

224. **Answer: C** - Loperimide (Imodium) is a piperidine derivative anti-diarrheal agent. It is used to treat chronic diarrhea, and it is contraindicated in acute diarrheas caused by *E coli, Salmonella* or *Shigella*.

225. **Answer: A** - Glipizide (Glucotrol) is sulfonylurea class hypoglycemic agent used to treat Type 2 diabetes mellitus (non-insulin-dependent diabetes mellitus; NIDDM). It is contraindicated in DKA.

226. **Answer: C** - Pioglitazone (Actos) is thiozolidinedione class hypoglycemic agent used to treat Type 2 diabetes mellitus (non-insulin-dependent diabetes mellitus; NIDDM). Its safety and efficacy have not been established in children.

227. **Answer: D** - Each statement is an accurate description of clinical trials.

228. **Answer: C** - Spironolactone, an aldosterone inhibitor and therefore a diuretic (K^+ sparing), has been associated with GI bleeds, breast cancer, metaolic acidosis and hyperkalemia. The other side effects listed are primarily associated with the use of the combined estrogen-progestin.

229. **Answer: B** - Ticlopidine (Ticlid) is a platelet aggregation inhibitor. GI and intracerebral hemorrhages and bone marrow depression are serious adverse reactions. Other adverse reactions include blood dyscrasias. Statement A is true of tirofian (Aggrastat), another platelet aggreagation inhibitor. Statements C and D are true of warfarin (Coumadin), a classic anticoagulant.

230. **Answer: B** - Zafirlukast is a leukotriene receptor antagonist used to treat asthma in adults and children over 12 years of age. Androstenedione is a precursor of testosterone and estrogens and is banned by the FDA. Cytomel is synthetic T3 and is used to treat hypothyroidism. Finasteride is a 5-alpha reductase inhibitor and is used in PCOS, BPH and treatment of male-pattern baldness.

231. **Answer: D** - Diabetes is defined as 2 or more fasting glucose levels greater than or equal to 126 mg/dL. Therefore, she should be directed to get a formal diagnosis and begin formal educational classes.

232. **Answer: D** - Granisetron (Kytril) is a $5HT_3$ receptor inhibitor used to treat the nausea and vomiting of chemotherapy/radiation therapy and post-operative nausea and vomiting. It is sometimes used in the nausea and vomiting of pregnancy. Butorphenol (Stadol) is a mixed opioid with analgesic properties and comes as a nasal spray. Tolcapone (Tasmar) is a catechol-O-methyltransferase (COMT) inhibitor and is used to treat Parkinson's disease. Topiramate (Topomax) blocks voltage dependent sodium channels and is used as an anti-seizure medication.

233. **Answer: D** - Answers A-C list the most common signs and symptoms of serotonin syndrome. Headaches, diarrhea and anorexia are not typically associated with serotonin syndrome.

234. **Answer: A** - All the statements are true.

235. **Answer: C** - *H. pylori* associated ulcers are treated with a PPI and antibiotics to decrease the acidity and eradicate the bacteria, respectively. The etiology of these ulcers indicates that neither a PPI or antibiotic alone is an effective treatment. OTC NSAIDs are often the cause of ulcers and/or exacerbators and should be avoided.

236. **Answer: C** - Hydrocortisone comes in many brand names. In addition to Cortef, Locoid and Westcort, it is marketed as Cortenema, Hydrocortone, A-hydroCort and Solu-Cortef. Inflixamab is marketed as Remicade and is an anti-rheumatic and anti-inflammatory agent used to treat RA and IBDs.

237. **Answer: C** - Infllixamab is a monoclonal antibody reacting with TNF-alpha. It is an anti-inflammatory but has immunosuppressive ahd hematopoietic effects as well. Hypersensitivity to the drug is relatively common and must be monitored. Creatine phosphokinase levels are more important in musculoskeletal disorders and generally do not need to be monitored in immunosuppressed patients.

238. **Answer: D** - Moxiflosacin is a quinolone anti-infective agent. Quinolones are contraindicated in an individual with a G6PD deficiency.

239. **Answer: A** - The "R" in the antineoplastic combination CHOP+R is for Rituxan, a monoclonal antibody, rituximab, which binds to the CD20 antigen on B cells. Ramelteon (Roserem) is a melatonin receptor agonist used tot treat insomnia. Ramipril (Altace) is an ACE inhibitor used to treat hypertension. Raloxiphene (Evista) is a non-steroidal SERM (selective estrogen receptor modulator). In CHOP+R, the "C" is for cyclophosphamide, "H" is for doxorubicin (hydroxydaunomycin antitumor antibiotic), "O" is for vincristine (Oncovin) and "P" is for presdnisone.

240. **Answer: A** - Metronidazole is the drug of choice against *Clostridium difficile* due to its lower price and good clinical efficacy. Clindamycin is ineffective against *Clostridia*, and *Clostridia* overgrowth is a serious potential adverse effect. Ketonidazole is an azole antifungal. Ciprofloxacin is fluroquinone without high efficacy against *Clostridium difficile.*

241. **Answer: A** - The "D" in the antineoplastic combination, DICE is for dexamethasone. Denileukin is an antineoplastic BRM (biological response modifier) but is not used in this combination. Desipramine is a TCA (tricyclic antidepressant), and diazepam is a benzodiazepine anxiolytic. In DICE, the "I" is for ifosfamide, "C" is for cisplatin and "E" is for etoposide.

242. **Answer: C** - Quinolones, NSAIDs and various food colorings should be avoided in patients with G6PD deficiency. The enzyme is found in red blood cells and protects against oxidative stress. G6PD has over 400 polymorphic variants. African Americans have some of the highest rates of polymorphism. This is believed to have developed as an evolutionary adaptation to malarial infection. There is no need to avoid Vitamin B_{12}.

243. **Answer: D** - All the chemotherapeutic agents are correctly paired with their mechanisms of action.

244. **Answer: B** - HIPAA does address patient privacy issues, and it is enforced by the Office of Civil Rights, not the Justice Department. Privacy is, in fact, one of its primary purposes. Statements II and IV are true.

245. **Answer: C** - Brompheniramine is a histamine antagonist (i.e. an anti-histamine) used for symptomatic relief of allergic and hypersensitivity reactions. Other adverse effects of brompheniramine include anemias and dyscrasias.

246. **Answer: B** - Diazepam and nateglinide do NOT induce photosensitivity in individuals. Naproxen and vinblastine do induce photoreactions. If a patient is photosensitive, it is important that they be informed which drugs may induce the reaction.

247. **Answer: B** - Chemical arachnoiditis (nausea, vomiting, headache, fever) is a primary side effect of intrathecal injection of cytarabine. Dexamethasone, co-administered, limits the effects of the arachnoiditis. There is no clear correlation between the rate of infusion and the appearance of the arachnoiditis.

248. **Answer: A** - N-acetylcysteine (Acetadote, Mucomyst, Mucosil) is a mucolytic cysteine derivative used in many UR conditions where there is excess mucus. It is also used as an antidote to acetaminophen overdose in both adults and children.

249. **Answer: D** - Pantoprazole (Protonix) is a PPI used to treat erosive esophagitis caused by GERD (gastroesophageal reflux disease). Filgrastim (Neupogen) is a leukocyte colony stimulating factor. Ondansetron (Zofran) is a 5HT3 antagonist. Atorvastatin (Lipitor) is an HMG-CoA reductase inhibitor.

250. **Answer: D** - All the statements are true in general of SERMs. Tamoxifen (Nolvadex) is a SERM used as an adjunct in breast cancer treatment and prevention in high-risk women. Other SERMs include clomiphene, fearelle, ormeloxifen, raloxifene and toremifine. They are also used to treat menopause, anovulation and osteoporosis. Ormeloxifene is used as a contraceptive. Bone pain is considered indicative of a positive response and should be managed with analgesics. Thromboembolic events occur more frequently in patients on all SERMs and must be monitored.

251. **Answer: C** - A bilateral orchiectomy and the use of an LH-RH antagonist are considered to be effective therapy for Stage III prostate cancer. Testosterone antagonists alone are not considered an effective therapy.

252. **Answer: B** - Fenofibrate is a fibric acid derivative and is used to decrease serum levels of LDL, total cholesterol, triglycerides and apolipoprotein B.

253. **Answer: C** - Alprazolam (Xanax) is a benzodiazepine anxiolytic. Finasteride (Proscar, Propecia, Fincar, Finpecia, Finax, Finast, Finara, Finalo, Prosteride, Gefina, Appecia) is an androgen inhibitor used in BPH and male-pattern baldness. Doxepin (Sinequan, Xepin, Zonalon) is a TCA (tricyclic antidepressant). Entacapone (Comtan) is a COMT inhibitor and an antidyskinetic. It is used to adjunctively treat Parkinson's disease.

254. **Answer: D** - Clozapine (Clozaril, Fazalco) is an **a**typical antipsychotic. Haloperidol (Haldol) is considered a typical antipsychotic. Temazepam (Restoril) is an anxiolytic. Guaifenesin (Mucinex, Robitussin) is an expectorant.

255. **Answer: D** - All the drugs listed except aripiprazole are used to treat tuberculosis. Aripiprazole is an antipsychotic and a neuroleptic used in the treatment of schizophrenia and bipolar disorder.

256. **Answer: C** - Diclofenac is a COX inhibitor marketed as Voltaren. Celecoxib is a COX-2 inhibitor and marketed as Celebrex. Propoxyphene is an opioid agonist marketed as Darvon. All three are used in the treatment of osteoarthritis. Guanfacine (Tenex) is a centrally acting anti-adrenergic agent used to treat hypertension.

257. **Answer: B** - Acetazolamide is a carbonic anhydrase inhibitor, increasing the excretion of sodium, potassium, bicarbonate and water. It can be used as a diuretic, an anti-glaucoma agent, an anti-convulsant, a urinary alkalzer and an agent to treat high-altitude sickness.

258. **Answer: D** - Methotrexate (MTX), Metronidazole (Flagyl) and Atorvastatin (Lipitor) are all Pregnancy category X medications; the use of contraception by women of reproductive age is required (FDA definition: "Adequate, well-controlled or observational studies in animals or pregnant women have demonstrated positive evidence of fetal abnormalities or risks. The use of the product is contraindicated in women who are or may become pregnant."). Loratadine (Alavert, Claritin) is a histamine$_1$-receptor antagonist used for seasonal allergies and is a Pregnancy Category B (FDA definition: "Animal studies have revealed no evidence of harm to the fetus, however, there are no adequate and well-controlled studies in pregnant women **OR** Animal studies have shown an adverse effect, but adequate and well-controlled studies in pregnant women have failed to demonstrate a risk to the fetus in any trimester.").

259. **Answer: A** - Ambien is the brand name used for zolpidem. Misoprostol is the generic name for Cytotec. Modafinil is sold as Provigil. Lisinopril is sold as Prinivil or Zestril.

260. **Answer: D** - Only statements I and II are correct. A Nuva Ring should be inserted monthly. NuvaRing contains both estrogens and progestins. Seasonale users take 84 active pills followed by 7 inactive pills, which allow for menses. Neither form of contraceptive gives any protection against STIs.

261. **Answer: C** - Miglitol is an alpha-glucosidease hypoglycemic agent used to treat Type 2 (non-insulin-dependent diabetes; NIDDM) and is contraindicated for Type 1 (insulin-dependent diabetes; IDDM).

262. **Answer: C** - Primidone is a barbiturate anti-convulsant and is used to treat seizure disorders. It is marketed as Mysoline. Prima is a made-up name. Plendil (felodipine) is a calcium channel blocker used to treat hypertension. Probalan is the brand name of probenecid, a sulfonamide-derived uricosuric used to treat gout.

263. **Answer: D** - Flumazenil is used as an antidote to benzodiazepines and acts as a competitive inhibitor at the GABA receptors. Nalmefene is a competitive antagonist at opioid receptors and is used in alcoholism treatment. Physostigmine is a classic acetylcholinesterase inhibitor and is used as an antidote for anticholinergics. Protamine is an anti-coagulant and complexes with heparin and neutralizes the anti-coagulative properties of both agents.

264. **Answer: B** - NSAIDs are contraindicated with any history of GI bleeding, as they are a major cause of ulcers.

265. **Answer: D** - Psyllium is a bulk laxative and is contraindicated with any intestinal obstruction or volvulus.

266. **Answer: D** - Testosterone is available in all the forms listed. Additionally, it is available as a transdermal patch.

267. **Answer: A** - An uncomfortable facial flushing is the most common side effect of niacin. Niacin is used to treat hyperlipidemia, pellagra and niacin deficiency.

268. **Answer: A** - Folvite is the brand name of folic acid. Bronchospasm is the only adverse effect listed that has been seen with Folvite use.

269. **Answer: D** - Statements II, III and IV are true. A1c does correlate with the lifespan of a red blood cell (rbc), but the lifespan of an rbc is on the order of 3-4 months (90-120 days), NOT 6-8 months. The other statements are true.

270. **Answer: D** - Tolterodine is an anti-cholinergic agent and is used as a urinary tract anti-spasmotic for patients with an overactive bladder.

271. **Answer: B** - Venlafaxine is an anti-depressant, and dosage listed is possible. Ezetimide is a cholesterol absorption inhibitor, and hydroxycobalamin is vitamin B_{12}. Nortriptyline IS an anti-depressent, but the dosage listed represents 1.2 g a day. Maximum dosage of Nortriptyline is 150 mg daily. All other dosages and routes for all the agents listed are possible.

Made in the USA
Monee, IL
10 September 2021